Curing
PMS
Naturally

with
Chinese
Medicine

Bob Flaws

BLUE POPPY PRESS

Published by:
BLUE POPPY PRESS, INC.
1775 LINDEN AVE.
BOULDER, CO 80304

First Edition, November, 1997

ISBN 0-936185-85-6   LC 97-71730
COPYRIGHT 1997 © BLUE POPPY PRESS

WARNING: When following some of the self-care techniques given in this book, failure to follow the author's instruction may result in side effects or negative reactions. Therefore, please be sure to follow the author's instructions carefully for all self-care techniques and modalities. For instance, wrong or excessive application of moxibustion may cause local burns with redness, inflammation, blistering, or even possible scarring. If you have any questions about doing these techniques safely and without unwanted side effects, please see a local professional practitioner for instruction.

DISCLAIMER: The information in this book is given in good faith. However, the author and the publishers cannot be held responsible for any error or omission. The publishers will not accept liabilities for any injuries or damages caused to the reader that may result from the reader's acting upon or using the content contained in this book.

COMP Designation: Original work using a standard translational terminology

Printed at Johnson's Printing in Boulder, CO
on essentially chlorine-free paper
Cover design by Jeff Fuller of Crescent Moon

10 9 8 7 6 5 4 3 2 1

Other books in this series include:

Curing Insomnia Naturally with Chinese Medicine
Curing Hay Fever Naturally with Chinese Medicine
Breast Health Naturally with Chinese Medicine
Curing Depression Naturally with Chinese Medicine
Curing Arthritis Naturally with Chinese Medicine

Preface

I have been practicing traditional Chinese medicine for almost 20 years, and for 17 of those years I have been specializing in Chinese medical gynecology. You could say that I have "written the book" (actually 10 or more) on all areas of Chinese gynecology in English. No matter what other gynecological diseases or complaints my patients may have, the vast majority also suffer from PMS. Based on my many years as a clinician, I can say without hesitation that traditional Chinese medicine treats premenstrual syndrome or PMS very well.

Although I have written numerous textbooks and clinical manuals for professionals on all aspects of Chinese gynecology, up till now, there has not been any simple discussion of the Chinese medical diagnosis and treatment of PMS written specifically for the lay reader. Therefore, I have created this book for sufferers of PMS and their friends and families. Hopefully, the reader will find that traditional Chinese medicine is an enlightening and empowering alternative or complement to more conventional treatment. Chinese medicine has a whole and holistic, centuries old, well developed and coherent theory about the cause and treatment of PMS. Not only is this theory enlightening, providing as it does a whole different perspective on this common complaint from modern Western medicine, it is also empowering. Based on this theory, women will find there are all sorts of things, most of which are free or very low cost, which they can do for themselves in order to relieve and even cure their PMS.

When I was a teenager, girls used to call their menstruation "the curse", as if PMS and menstrual pain were simply the lot of all Eve's daughters. Chinese medicine says that this is not so. PMS does not need to occur, and if it does, Chinese medicine has ways to eliminate or minimize it.

Bob Flaws
Boulder, CO
March 1997

Table of Contents

Introduction

Denise was not a happy camper. She had been cranky and irritable for several days. She was snappish with her boyfriend and found herself in tears over the littlest of things. Partly, she was angry at herself for being so out of control. Her life was not all that bad. When her boyfriend had reluctantly asked her if she was going to get her period in the next couple of days, she had really lost her top. They had had a big argument and he had walked out, slamming the door behind him. When he came back, he walked around the apartment as if on eggshells. This only infuriated Denise all the more. Three days later, Denise did, in fact, get her period. The next month, the same thing or some minor variation happened all over again.

Sound familiar? If so, this book many very well help you break the cycle of PMS. According to traditional Chinese medicine, PMS is most definitely classified as a valid gynecological complaint or disease. The good news is that Chinese doctors (including acupuncturists) have been curing women's PMS for centuries if not millennia.

This book is a layperson's guide to the diagnosis and treatment of PMS with Chinese medicine. In it, you will learn what causes PMS *and what you can do about it*. Hopefully, you will be able to identify yourself and your symptoms in these pages. If you can see yourself in the signs and symptoms I discuss below, I feel confident I will be able to share with you a number of self-help techniques which can minimize your monthly discomfort. I have been specializing in the Chinese medical treatment of gyne-cological complaints for 17 years, and I have helped hundreds of

Western women cure or relieve their PMS. Chinese medicine cannot cure every gynecological disease, but when it comes to PMS, Chinese medicine is the best alternative I know. When a woman calls me and says that PMS is her major complaint, I know that, if she follows my advice, together we can cure or at least reduce her premenstrual signs and symptoms.

What is PMS?

According to *The Merck Manual*, PMS is a "condition characterized by nervousness, irritability, emotional instability, depression, and possibly headaches, edema, and mastalgia;[1] it occurs seven to ten days before menstruation and disappears a few hours after the onset of menstrual flow."[2] When nervousness, irritability, depression, and emotional instability or lability are the main symptoms, this disease is also referred to as PMT, premenstrual tension, and PMDD, premenstrual dysphoric disorder. In actual clinical fact, the list of accompanying signs and symptoms is much longer than the one presented above. As we will see below, some women's PMS includes dozens of symptoms and complaints. In fact, more than 150 symptoms have been reported in the Western medical literature in association with PMS.[3] It is also true that, although the authors of *The Merck Manual* say PMS begins seven to ten days before each menses, in some women it may begin two weeks or more before each period. Though the symptoms of PMS vary from woman to woman, they do occur during a specific and relatively constant time of the menstrual cycle and have a clear beginning and end.

---

[1] Mastalgia means breast pain.

[2] *The Merck Manual of Diagnosis & Therapy*, Robert Berkow, MD, editor, Merck, Sharp & Dohme Research Laboratories, Rahway, NJ, 1987, p. 1710

[3] *Premenstrual Syndrome (PMS)*, www.dash.com/netro/nwxtmr/tmr0196 /pms. html

Is PMS really a disease?

When PMS first entered the public's consciousness in the 1970s, there was some controversy over whether it was a "real" disease. Other people wondered if PMS was a "new" disease. In actual fact, PMS was first identified as a Western medical entity in 1931. Obviously, the editors and authors of *The Merck Manual* consider this a legitimate disease simply by its inclusion in their popular and widely used clinical reference, and Chinese doctors have known for 1,000 years or more that some women get certain symptoms cyclically before each menses. Recent studies have established that premenstrual changes, both psychological and physical, are organically based.[4] This means that the signs and symptoms of PMS are related to chemical changes that occur in the body in the time before the onset of the monthly menstruation. As a clinician, I can assure women that PMS is very much a "real" complaint and that it is not just a fabrication of one's mind, although, as we will see below, the mind most certainly does play an important part in this condition's cause and treatment.

Up to 80% of women of reproductive age experience premenstrual emotional and physical changes. It is estimated that 20-40% of these women experience some difficulty as a result of these changes during their premenstruum and 2.5-5% of sufferers report a significant negative impact on their work, lifestyle, or relationships.

At the moment, there is no clinical or laboratory test to document a diagnosis of PMS. Rather, its diagnosis depends on the use of a menstrual calendar to track and verify the fact that a woman's signs and symptoms are definitely related to her menstrual cycle month after month.

---

[4] *Premenstrual Syndrome*, www.medhlp.netusa.net/general/womens/pms.txt

What causes PMS?

Modern Western medicine has yet to identify all the biological mechanisms of all the symptoms of PMS. However, many of the most prominent symptoms of PMS have to do with fluctuations in estrogen and progesterone production. Estrogen and progesterone are the two main hormones secreted by the ovaries which control the menstrual cycle. Estrogen exerts a fluid-retaining action on body tissues, and fluid retention plays a part in such PMS symptoms as weight gain, edema, abdominal bloating, and breast tenderness and pain. Therefore, some Western clinicians refer to PMS as a hyperestrogenosis condition, meaning too much production of estrogen. Other Western clinicians focus more on a progesterone insufficiency which then makes estrogen production appear *relatively* excessive.

It has also been suggested that PMS is due to a vitamin B_6 deficiency, low blood sugar, and/or a high level of prolactin, the hormone which governs milk production. Unfortunately, none of these theories account for all the various symptoms of PMS. Another recent theory holds that PMS is caused by sudden changes in the levels of naturally occurring morphine-like substances in the brain. According to this theory, cyclical changes in female hormone levels produce fluctuations in the levels of these morphine-like substances in the brain. First, a rise in these substances causes depression for a week to 10 days before menstruation, and then their sudden drop just before the onset of menstruation leads to nervousness and irritability. At the moment, this theory also does not explain all the signs and symptoms of PMS.

However, no matter whether estrogen is truly excess or only seemingly so due to a progesterone insufficiency, three questions remain about the causes of PMS according to Western medicine: 1) Why are these hormones out of balance in some women and are not in others? 2) What are the mechanisms at work in the symptoms not due to an excess of estrogen? And 3) what can a

4

woman do about any of this? Likewise, why do only certain women have a B_6 deficiency, why do only some women's brains over secrete morphine-like substances, and what can a woman do to prevent and change these things?

How Western medicine treats PMS

When Western MDs try to treat PMS, they usually do so using a combination of diet and lifestyle changes coupled with a prescription for one or more Western pharmaceuticals. There are three main pharmaceutical approaches to PMS. The first is diuretics. If many of the symptoms of PMS are due to water retention, then giving diuretics to evacuate this retained water through urination should make those symptoms better. Secondly, if this condition is due to abnormal levels of estrogen and progesterone, than trying to manipulate these levels externally also makes sense. Thus Western MDs may prescribe natural progesterone supplementation, artificial progesterone, called progestin, or oral contraceptives, *i.e,.* birth control pills. And third, given that many of the most upsetting premenstrual symptoms are mental-emotional, some Western MDs resort to prescribing tranquilizers and antidepressants to deal with nervousness, anxiety, and depression.

Unfortunately, many women experience side effects from any or all of these three types of Western medication. According to James W. Long, MD, author of *The Essential Guide to Prescription Drugs*, hydrochlorothiazide, the diuretic suggested by the authors of *The Merck Manual*, may cause skin rashes, hives, headache, blurred or yellowed vision, indigestion, nausea, vomiting, diarrhea, fatigue, weakness, fever, sore throat, and abnormal bleeding or bruising, not to mention decrease in sex drive in 12% of patients who take it.[5] Likewise, oral birth control pills may cause skin rashes, hives, headache, nervous tension, irritability, nausea,

---

[5] Long, James W., *The Essential Guide to Prescription Drugs*, Harper & Row, NY, 1990, p. 527

5

vomiting, bloating, and diarrhea, many of the same symptoms which some PMS sufferers actually complain of. In addition, birth control pills can also cause thrombophlebitis, pulmonary embolism, stroke, or heart attack.[6] Diazepam, more commonly known as Valium, is the tranquilizer *The Merck Manual* recommends for PMS. Dr. Long lists the potential side effects of Valium as rashes and hives, dizziness, fainting, blurred and double vision, slurred speech, nausea, sweating, and even, paradoxically, excitement, agitation, anger, and rage.[7] In addition, Prozac and Zoloft, commonly prescribed antidepressants classified as selective serotonin reuptake inhibitors (SSRIs), are also prescribed for some women's PMS. The potential side effects of Prozac include hives, rashes, itching, headache, nervousness, insomnia, drowsiness, tremors, dizziness, fatigue, impaired concentration, altered taste, nausea, vomiting, and diarrhea.[8] Thus many women cannot take or do not want to take these types of Western pharmaceuticals.

Happily, many Western clinicians do recognize that diet and lifestyle play a part in the cause, treatment, and prevention of PMS. In terms of diet, Western MDs typically counsel PMS sufferers to reduce salt consumption since sodium can cause water retention. In addition, women are told to increase protein and decrease sugar consumption. Many women are also recommended to take a B vitamin supplement (especially B_6) and increased magnesium. We will look at sugar and salt from the Chinese perspective below. Basically, Chinese doctors agree with these dietary recommendations but make even more precise and extensive ones, fine tuning each woman's diet to uniquely fit her.

In terms of lifestyle, many Western clinicians today also realize that there is a pyschosomatic component to PMS. Psychosomatic

---

[6] *Ibid.*, p. 719

[7] *Ibid.*, p. 393

[8] *Ibid.*, p. 481

6

does not mean a disease is just in one's head. It means that there is a mutual relationship between one's body and one's mind. Bodily functions affect what the mind thinks and feels. Vice versa, what one thinks and feels also affects the body's functions. Therefore, some MDs will also recommend counseling and/or various types of stress reduction, and we will also talk about these from the Chinese point of view. However, although proper diet and lifestyle can eliminate mild to moderate PMS, they are seldom sufficient by themselves to eliminate moderate to severe PMS. Therefore, for many women, proper diet and counseling or stress reduction are not enough.

Western medicine, by its own admission, has no cure for PMS.[9] The best it has to offer at the present time is a collection of treatments meant to alleviate the symptoms of PMS. Happily, since Chinese medicine does cure PMS *without side effects*, it does offer a safe and effective alternative to the types of pharmaceuticals discussed above.[10]

East is East and West is West

In order for the reader to understand and make sense of the rest of this book on Chinese medicine and PMS, one must understand that Chinese medicine is a distinct and separate system of medical thought and practice from modern Western medicine. This means that one must shift models of reality when it comes to thinking about Chinese medicine. It has taken the Chinese more than 2,000 years to develop this medical system. In fact, Chinese

---

[9] "How to Find Out if You Have PMS", *The Virtual Hospital, Iowa Health Book*, www.indy.radiology.uiowa.edu/Patients/IHB/Family Practice/ AFP/ November/NovThree.html

[10] As of this writing, there is research being carried on assessing the beneficial effects of melatonin supplementation and treating PMS with light therapy. In my experience, a common side effect of melatonin is profuse and disturbing dreams and even nightmares. As we will see below, light or sunlight therapy does make sense from the Chinese medical point of view.

7

medicine is the oldest continually practiced, literate, professional medicine in the world. As such one cannot understand Chinese medicine by trying to explain it in Western scientific or medical terms.

Most people reading this book have probably taken high school biology back when they were sophomores. Whether we recognize it or not, most of us Westerners think of what we learned about the human body in high school as "the really real" description of reality, not one possible description. However, if Chinese medicine is to make any sense to Westerners at all, one must be able to entertain the notion that there are potentially other valid descriptions of the human body, its functions, health, and disease. In grappling with this fundamentally important issue, it is useful to think about the concepts of a map and the terrain it describes.

If we take the United States of America as an example, we can have numerous different maps of this country's land mass. One map might show population. Another might show per capita incomes. Another might show religious or ethnic distributions. Yet another might be a road map. And still another might be a map showing political, *i.e.*, state boundaries. In fact, there could be an infinite number of potentially different maps of the United States depending on what one was trying to show and do. As long as the map is based on accurate information and has been created with self-consistent logic, then one map is not necessarily more correct than another. The issue is to use the right map for what you are trying to do. If one wants to drive from Chicago to Washington, DC, then a road map is probably the right one *for that job* but is not necessarily a truer or "more real" description of the United States than a map showing annual rainfall.

What I am getting at here is that *the map is not the terrain.* The Western biological map of the human body is only one potentially useful medical map. It is no more true than the traditional Chinese medical map, and the "facts" of one map cannot be reduced to the criteria or standards of another *unless they share the same logic right from the beginning.* As long as the Western medical map is capable of solving a person's disease in a cost-effective, time-efficient manner without side effects or iatrogenesis (meaning doctor-caused disease), then it is a useful map. Chinese medicine needs to be judged in the same way. The Chinese medical map of health and disease is just as "real" as the Western biological map as long as by using it professional practitioners are able to solve their patients' health problems in a safe and effective way.

Therefore, the following chapter is an introduction to the basics of Chinese medicine. Unless one understands some of the fundamental theories and "facts" of Chinese medicine, one will not be able to understand or accept the reasons for some of the Chinese medical treatments of PMS. As the reader will quickly see from this brief overview of Chinese medicine, "This doesn't look like Kansas, Toto!"

An Overview of the Chinese Medical Map

In this chapter, we will look at an overview of Chinese medicine. In particular, we will discuss yin and yang, qi, blood, and essence, the viscera and bowels, and the channels and network vessels. Then, in the following chapter, we will go on to see how Chinese medicine views the menstual cycle and menstruation itself. After that, we will look at the Chinese medical diagnosis and treatment of a wide range of premenstrual signs and symptoms.

Yin & Yang

To understand Chinese medicine, one must first understand the concepts of yin and yang since these are the most basic concepts in this system. Yin and yang are the cornerstones for understanding, diagnosing, and treating the body and mind in Chinese medicine. In a sense, all the other theories and concepts of Chinese medicine are nothing other than an elaboration of yin and yang. Most people have probably already heard of yin and yang but may have only a fuzzy idea of what these terms mean.

The concepts of yin and yang can be used to describe everything that exists in the universe, including all the parts and functions of the body. Originally, yin referred to the shady side of a hill and yang to the sunny side of the hill. Since sunshine and shade are two, interdependent sides of a single reality, these two aspects of the hill are seen as part of a single whole. Other examples of yin and yang are that night exists only in relation to day and cold exists only in relation to heat. According to Chinese thought,

11

every single thing that exists in the universe has these two aspects, a yin and a yang. Thus everything has a front and a back, a top and a bottom, a left and a right, and a beginning and an end. However, a thing is yin or yang *only in relation to its paired complement*. Nothing is in itself yin or yang.

It is the concepts of yin and yang which make Chinese medicine a holistic medicine. This is because, based on this unitary and complementary vision of reality, no body part or body function is viewed as separate or isolated from the whole person. The table below shows a partial list of yin and yang pairs as they apply to

Yin	Yang
form	function
organs	bowels
blood	qi
inside	outside
front of body	back of body
right side	left side
lower body	upper body
cool, cold	warm, hot
stillness	activity, movement

the body. However, it is important to remember that each item listed is either yin or yang only in relation to its complementary partner. Nothing is absolutely and all by itself either yin or yang. As we can see from the above list, it is possible to describe every aspect of the body in terms of yin and yang.

Qi

Qi (pronounced chee) and blood are the two most important complementary pairs of yin and yang within the human body. It is said that, in the world, yin and yang are water and fire, but in the human body, yin and yang are blood and qi. Qi is yang in relation to blood which is yin. Qi is often translated as energy and certainly energy is a manifestation of qi. Chinese language scholars would say, however, that qi is larger than any single type of energy described by modern Western science. Paul Unschuld, perhaps the greatest living sinologist, translates the word qi as influences. This conveys the sense that qi is what is responsible for change and movement. Thus, within Chinese medicine, qi is that which motivates all movement and transformation or change.

In Chinese medicine, qi is defined as having five specific functions:

1. Defense

It is qi which is responsible for protecting the exterior of the body from invasion by external pathogens. This qi, called defensive qi, flows through the exterior portion of the body.

2. Transformation

Qi transforms substances so that they can be utilized by the body. An example of this function is the transformation of the food we eat into nutrients to nourish the body, thus producing more qi and blood.

3. Warming

Qi, being relatively yang, is inherently warm and one of the main functions of the qi is to warm the entire body, both inside and out. If this warming function of the qi is weak, cold may cause the flow of qi and blood to be congealed similar to cold's effect on water producing ice.

13

4. Restraint

It is qi which holds all the organs and substances in their proper place. Thus all the organs, blood, and fluids need qi to keep them from falling or leaking out of their specific pathways. If this function of the qi is weak, then problems like uterine prolapse, easy bruising, or urinary incontinence may occur.

5. Transportation

Qi provides the motivating force for all transportation and movement in the body. Every aspect of the body that moves is moved by the qi. Hence the qi moves the blood and body fluids throughout the body. It moves food through the stomach and blood through the vessels.

Blood

In Chinese medicine, blood refers to the red fluid that flows through our vessels the same as in modern Western medicine, but it also has meanings and implications which are different from those in modern Western medicine. Most basically, blood is that substance which nourishes and moistens all the body tissues. Without blood, no body tissue can function properly. In addition, when blood is insufficient or scanty, tissue becomes dry and withers.

Qi and blood are closely interrelated. It is said that, "Qi is the commander of the blood and blood is the mother of qi." This means that it is qi which moves the blood but that it is the blood which provides the nourishment and physical foundation for the creation and existence of the qi.

In Chinese medicine, blood provides the following functions for the body:

1. Nourishment

Blood nourishes the body. Along with qi, the blood goes to every part of the body. When the blood is insufficient, function decreases and tissue atrophies or shrinks.

2. Moistening

Blood moistens the body tissues. This includes the skin, eyes, and ligaments and tendons or what are simply called the sinews of the body in Chinese medicine. Thus blood insufficiency can cause drying out and consequent stiffening of various body tissues throughout the body.

3. Blood provides the material foundation for the spirit or mind.

In Chinese medicine, the mind and body are not two separate things. The spirit is nothing other than a great accumulation of qi. The blood (yin) supplies the material support and nourishment for the spirit (yang) so that it accumulates, becomes bright (*i.e.*, conscious and clever), and stays rooted in the body. If the blood becomes insufficient, the mind can "float," causing problems like insomnia, agitation, and unrest.

Essence

Along with qi and blood, essence is one of the three most important constituents of the body. Essence is the most fundamental, essential material the body utilizes for its growth, maturation, and reproduction. There are two forms of this essence. We inherit essence from our parents and we also produce our own essence from the food we eat, the liquids we drink, and the air we breathe.

The essence which comes from our parents is what determines our basic constitution, strength, and vitality. We each have a finite, limited amount of this inherited essence. It is important to protect and conserve this essence because all bodily functions depend upon it, and, when it is gone, we die. Thus the depletion of essence has serious implications for our overall health and well-being. Happily, the essence derived from food and drink helps to bolster and support this inherited essence. Thus, if we eat well and do not consume more qi and blood than we create each day, then when we sleep at night, this surplus qi and more especially blood is transformed into essence.

The Viscera & Bowels

In Chinese medicine, the internal organs (called viscera so as not to become confused with the Western biological entities of the same name) have a wider area of function and influence than in Western medicine. Each viscus has distinct responsibilities for maintaining the physical and psychological health of the individual. When thinking about the internal viscera according to Chinese medicine, it is more accurate to view them as spheres of influence or a network that spreads throughout the body, rather than as a distinct and separate physical organ as described by Western science. This is why the famous German sinologist, Manfred Porkert, refers to them as orbs rather than as organs. In Chinese medicine, the relationship between the various viscera and other parts of the body is made possible by the channel and network vessel system which we will discuss below.

In Chinese medicine, there are five main viscera which are relatively yin and six main bowels which are relatively yang. The five yin viscera are the heart, lungs, liver, spleen, and kidneys. The six yang bowels are the stomach, small intestine, large intestine, gallbladder, urinary bladder, and a system that Chinese medicine refers to as the triple burner. All the functions of the entire body are subsumed or described under these eleven organs or spheres of influence. Thus Chinese medicine *as a system* does not have a pancreas, a pituitary gland, or the ovaries. None-theless, all the functions of these Western organs are described under the Chinese medical system of the five viscera and six bowels.

Within this system, the five viscera are the most important. These are the organs that Chinese medicine says are responsible for the creation and transformation of qi and blood and the storage of essence. For instance, the kidneys are responsible for the excretion of urine but are also responsible for hearing, the strength of the bones, sex, reproduction, maturation and growth, the lower and upper back, and the lower legs in general and the knees in particular.

Visceral Correspondences

Organ	Tissue	Sense	Spirit	Emotion
Kidneys	bones/ head hair	hearing	will	fear
Liver	sinews	sight	ethereal soul	anger
Spleen	flesh	taste	thought	thinking/ worry
Lungs	skin/body hair	smell	corporeal soul	grief/ sadness
Heart	blood vessels	speech	spirit	joy/fright

This points out that the Chinese viscera may have the same name and even some overlapping functions but yet are quite different from the organs of modern Western medicine. Each of the five Chinese medical viscera also has a corresponding tissue, sense, spirit, and emotion related to it. These are outlined in the table above.

In addition, each Chinese medical viscus or bowel possesses both a yin and a yang aspect. The yin aspect of a viscus or bowel refers

17

to its substantial nature or tangible form. Further, an organ's yin is responsible for the nurturing, cooling, and moistening of that viscus or bowel. The yang aspect of the viscus or bowel represents its functional activities or what it does. An organ's yang aspect is also warming. These two aspects, yin and yang, form and function, cooling and heating, when balanced create good health. However, if either yin or yang becomes too strong or too weak, the result will be disease.

The kidneys

In Chinese medicine, the kidneys are considered to be the foundation of our life. Because the developing fetus looks like a large kidney and because the kidneys are the main viscus for the storage of inherited essence, the kidneys are referred to as the prenatal root. Thus keeping the kidney qi strong and kidney yin and yang in relative balance is considered essential to good health and longevity. The basic Chinese medical statements of fact about the the kidneys are:

1. The kidneys are considered responsible for human reproduction, development, and maturation.

These are the same functions we used when describing the essence. This is because the essence is stored in the kidneys. Health problems related to reproduction, development, and maturation are considered to be problems of the kidney essence. Excessive sexual activity, drug use, or simple prolonged over-exhaustion can all damage and consume kidney essence. Kidney essence is also consumed by the simple act of aging.

2. The kidneys are the foundation of water metabolism.

The kidneys work in coordination with the lungs and spleen to insure that water is spread properly throughout the body and that excess water is excreted as urination. Therefore, problems such as edema, excessive dryness, or excessive day or nighttime urination can indicate a weakness of kidney function.

3. The kidneys are responsible for hearing since the kidneys open through the portals of the ears.

Therefore, auditory problems such as diminished hearing and ringing in the ears can be due to kidney weakness.

5. The kidneys rule the grasping of qi.

This means that one of the functions of the kidney qi is to pull down or absorb the breath from the lungs and root it in the lower abdomen. Certain types of asthma and chronic cough are the result of a weakness in this kidney function.

6. The kidneys rule the bones and marrow.

This means that problems of the bones, such as osteoporosis, degenerative disc disease, and weak legs and knees, can all reflect a kidney problem.

7. Kidney yin and yang are the foundation for the yin and yang of all the other organs and bowels and body tissues of the entire body.

This is another way of saying that the kidneys are the foundation of our life. If either kidney yin or yang is insufficient, eventually the yin or yang of the other organs will also become insufficient.

8. The kidneys store the will.

If kidney qi is insufficient, this aspect of our human nature can be weakened. Conversely, pushing ourselves to extremes, such as long distance running or cycling, can eventually exhaust our kidneys.

9. Fear is the emotion associated with the kidneys.

This means that fear can manifest when the kidney qi is insufficient. Vice versa, constant or excessive fear can damage the kidneys and make them weak.

10. The low back is the mansion of the kidneys.

This means that, of all the areas of the body, the low back is the most closely related to the health of the kidneys. If the kidneys are weak, then there may be low back pain. It is because of this and the fact that the kidneys are associated with the bones that the kidneys are the first and most important viscus in terms of the health and well-being of the low back according to Chinese medicine.

The liver

In Chinese medicine, the liver is associated with one's emotional state, with digestion, and with menstruation in women. As we will see in the following chapters, the liver is the lynchpin in the Chinese medical diagnosis and treatment of PMS. The basic Chinese medical statements of facts concerning the liver include:

1. The liver controls coursing and discharge.

Coursing and discharge refer to the uninhibited spreading of qi to every part of the body. If the liver is not able to maintain the free and smooth flow of qi throughout the body, multiple physical and emotional symptoms can develop. This function of the liver is most easily damaged by emotional causes and, in particular, by anger and frustration. For example, if the liver is stressed due to pent-up anger, the flow of liver qi can become depressed or stagnate.

Liver qi stagnation can cause a wide range of health problems, including PMS, chronic digestive disturbance, depression, and low back pain. Therefore, it is essential to keep our liver qi flowing freely.

2. The liver stores the blood.

This means that the liver regulates the amount of blood in circulation. In particular, when the body is at rest, the blood in the extremities returns to the liver. As an extension of this, it is said in Chinese medicine that the liver is yin in form but yang in function. Thus the liver requires sufficient blood to keep it *and its associated tissues* moist and supple, cool and relaxed.

3. The liver controls the sinews.

The sinews refer mainly to the tendons and ligaments in the body. Proper function of the tendons and ligaments depends upon the nourishment of liver blood to keep them moist and supple.

4. The liver opens into the portals of the eyes.

The eyes are the specific sense organ corresponding to the liver. Therefore, many eye problems are related to the liver in Chinese medicine.

5. The emotion associated with the liver is anger.

Anger is the emotion that typically arises when the liver is diseased and especially when its qi does not flow freely. Conversely, anger damages the liver. Thus the emotions related to the stagnation of qi in the liver are frustration, anger, and rage.

The heart

Although the heart is the emperor of the body–mind according to Chinese medicine, it does not play as large a role in the creation and treatment of disease as one might think. Rather than the emperor initiating the cause of disease, in Chinese medicine, mostly enduring disease eventually affects the heart. Especially

21

in terms of PMS, disturbances of the heart tend to be secondary rather than primary. By this I mean that first some other viscus or bowel becomes diseased and then the heart feels the negative effect. The basic statements of fact about the heart in Chinese medicine are:

1. The heart governs the blood.

This means that it is the heart qi which "stirs" or moves the blood within its vessels. This is roughly analogous to the heart's pumping the blood in Western medicine. The pulsation of the blood through the arteries due to the contraction of the heart is referred to as the "stirring of the pulse." In fact, the Chinese word for pulse and vessel is the same. So this could also be translated as the "stirring of the vessels."

2. The heart stores the spirit.

The spirit refers to the mind in Chinese medicine. Therefore, this statement underscores that mental function, mental clarity, and mental equilibrium are all associated with the heart. If the heart does not receive enough qi or blood or if the heart is disturbed by something, the spirit may become restless and this may produce symptoms of mental-emotional unrest, heart palpitations, insomnia, profuse dreams, etc.

3. The heart governs the vessels.

This statement is very close to number one above. The vessels refer to the blood vessels and also to the pulse.

4. The heart governs speech.

If heart function becomes abnormal, this may be reflected in various speech problems and especially in raving and delirious speech, muttering to oneself, and speaking incoherently.

5. The heart opens into the portal of the tongue.

Because the heart has a special relationship with the tip of the tongue, heart problems may manifest as sores on the tip of the tongue.

6. Joy is the emotion associated with the heart.

The word joy has been interpreted by both Chinese and Westerners in different ways. On the one hand, joy can mean overexcitation, in which case excessive joy can cause problems with the Chinese medical functions of the heart in terms of governing the blood and storing the spirit. On the other hand, joy may be seen as an antidote to the other six emotions of Chinese medicine. From this point of view, joy causes the flow of qi (and therefore blood) to relax and become more moderate and harmonious. If some other emotion causes the qi to become bound or move chaotically, then joy can make it relax and flow normally and smoothly.

The spleen

The spleen is less important in Western medicine than it is in Chinese medicine. Since at least the Yuan dynasty (1280-1368 CE), the spleen has been one of the two most important viscera of Chinese medicine (the other being the kidneys). In Chinese medicine, the spleen plays a pivotal role in the creation of qi and blood and in the circulation and transfomation of body fluids. Therefore, when it comes to the spleen, it is especially important not to think of this Chinese viscus in the same way as the Western spleen. The main statements of fact concerning the spleen in Chinese medicine are:

1. The spleen governs movement and transformation.

This refers to the movement and transformation of foods and liquids through the digestive system. In this case, movement and transformation may be paraphrased as digestion. However, secondarily, movement and transformation also refer to the movement and transformation of body fluids through the body. It is the spleen qi which is largely responsible for controlling liquid metabolism in the body.

2. The spleen restrains the blood.

As mentioned above, one of the five functions of the qi is to restrain the fluids of the body, including the blood, within their proper channels and reservoirs. If the spleen qi is healthy and abundant, then the blood is held within its vessels properly. However, if the spleen qi becomes weak and insufficient, then the blood may flow outside its channels and vessels resulting in various types of pathological bleeding. This includes various types of pathological bleeding associated with the menstrual cycle.

3. The spleen stores the constructive.

The constructive is one of the types of qi in the body. Specifically, it is the qi responsible for nourishing and constructing the body and its tissues. This constructive qi is closely associated with the process of digestion and the creation of qi and blood out of food and liquids. If the spleen fails to store or runs out of constructive qi, then the person becomes hungry on the one hand, and eventually becomes fatigued on the other.

4. The spleen governs the muscles and flesh.

This statement is closely allied to the previous one. It is the constructive qi which constructs or nourishes the muscles and flesh. If there is sufficient spleen qi producing sufficient constructive qi, then the person's body is well fleshed and rounded. In addition, their muscles are normally strong. Conversely, if the spleen becomes weak, this may lead to emaciation and/or lack of strength.

5. The spleen governs the four limbs.

This means that the strength and function of the four limbs is closely associated with the spleen. If the spleen is healthy and strong, then there is sufficient strength in the four limbs and warmth in the four extremities. If the spleen becomes weak and insufficient, then there may be lack of strength in the four limbs, lack of warmth in the extremities, or even tingling and numbness in the extremities.

6. The spleen opens into the portal of the mouth.

Just as the ears are the portals of the kidneys, the eyes are the portal of the liver, and the tongue is the portal of the heart, the mouth is the portal of the spleen. Therefore, spleen disease often manifests as mouth or canker sores or bleeding from the gums.

7. Thought is the emotion associated with the spleen.

In the West, we do not usually think of thought as an emotion per se. Be that as it may, in Chinese medicine it is classified along with anger, joy, fear, fright, grief, and melancholy. In particular, thinking, or perhaps I should say overthinking, causes the spleen qi to bind. This means that the spleen qi does not flow harmoniously and this typically manifests as loss of appetite, abdominal bloating after meals, and indigestion.

8. The spleen is the source of engenderment and transformation.

Engenderment and transformation refer to the creation or production of the qi and blood out of the food and drink we take in each day. If the spleen recieves adequate food and drink and then properly transforms that food and drink, it engenders or creates the qi and blood. Although the kidneys and lungs also participate in the creation of the qi, while the kidneys and heart also participate in the creation of the blood, the spleen is the pivotal viscus in both processes, and spleen qi weakness and insufficiency is a leading cause of qi and blood insufficiency and weakness.

The lungs

The lungs are not one of the main Chinese viscera in the cause of PMS. However, like the heart, the lungs often bear the brunt of disease processes initiated in other viscera and bowels. As in Western medicine, the lungs are often subject to externally invading pathogens resulting in respiratory tract diseases. However, the lungs sphere of influence also includes the skin and fluid metabolism. The main statements of fact regarding the lungs in Chinese medicine are:

1. The lungs govern the qi.

Specifically, the lungs govern the downward spread and circulation of the qi. It is the lung qi which moves all the rest of the qi in the body out to the edges and from the top of the body downward. Thus the lung qi is something like a sprinkler spraying out qi. As an extension of this, this downward qi then makes sure body fluids are moved throughout the body and eventually down to the kidneys and bladder and, eventually, out of the body.

2. The lungs govern the skin and hair.

The skin and body hair correspond with the lungs. If the lungs become diseased, this often manifests as skin problems.

3. The lungs govern the voice.

If there is sufficient lung qi, the voice is strong and clear. If there is insufficient lung qi, then the voice is weak and the person tries not to speak as a way of conserving their energy.

26

4. The lungs govern the free flow and regulation of the water passageways.

This statement empahsizes the lung qi's role in moving body fluids outward and downward throughout the body, ultimately to arrive at the urinary bladder. If the lung qi fails to maintain the free flow and regulation of the water passageways, then fluids will collect and transform into dampness, thus producing water swelling or edema.

5. The lungs govern the defensive exterior.

We say above that the qi defends the body against invasion by external pathogens. In Chinese medicine, the exterior–most layer of the body is the area where the defensive qi circulates and the place where this defense, therefore, takes place. In particular, it is the lungs which govern this defensive qi. If the lungs function normally and there is sufficient defensive qi, then the body cannot be invaded by external pathogens. If the lungs are weak and the defensive qi is insufficient, then external pathogens may easily invade the exterior of the body, causing complaints such as colds, flus, and allergies.

6. The lungs are the florid canopy.

This means that the lungs are like a tent spreading over the top of all the other viscera and bowels. On the one hand, they are the first viscus to be assaulted by external pathogens invading the body from the top. On the other, any pathogenic qi moving upward in the body eventually may accumulate in and affect the lungs.

7. The lungs are the delicate viscus.

Because the lungs are the most delicate of all the viscera and bowels, they are the most easily invaded by external pathogens. This is the Chinese explanation for the prevalence of colds and flus in comparison to other types of diseases.

8. The lungs form snivel.

This means that snivel or nasal mucus has to do, at least in part, with lung function. If the lungs are functioning correctly, there should not be any runny nose or nasal congestion.

9. The lungs open into the portal of the nose.

This statement is similar to the one above. However, it approaches the issue from a slightly different perspective. The implication of this statement is that diseases having to do with the nose and its function are often associated with the Chinese medical idea of the lungs.

Because the viscera are relatively more important than the bowels in Chinese medicine, I will not take up the space here to enumerate all the functions of each bowel. Suffice it to say that each viscus is paired with a bowel in a yin-yang relationship. The kidneys are paired with the urinary bladder, the liver is paired with the gallbladder, the heart is paired with the small intestine, the spleen is paired with the stomach, and the lungs are paired with the large intestine. In the case of the urinary bladder, gallbladder, and stomach, these bowels receive their qi from their paired viscus and function very much as an extension of that viscus. The relationship between the other two viscera and bowels is not as close.

Above I mentioned that there are five viscera and six bowels. The sixth bowel is called the triple burner. It is said in Chinese that, "The triple burner has a function but no form." The name triple burner refers to the three main areas of the torso. The upper burner is the chest. The middle burner is the space from the bottom of the rib cage to the level of the navel. The lower burner is the lower abdomen below the navel. These three spaces are called burners because all of the functions and transformations of the viscera and bowels which they contain are "warm" transformations similar to food cooking in a pot on a stove or similar to an alchemical transformation in a furnace. In fact, the

28

triple burner is nothing other than a generalized concept of how the other viscera and bowels function together as an organic unit in terms of the digestion of foods and liquids and the circulation and transformation of body fluids.

The Channels & Network Vessels

Each viscus and bowel has a corresponding channel with which it is connected. In Chinese medicine, the inside of the body is made up of the viscera and bowels. The outside of the body is composed of the sinews and bones, muscles and flesh, and skin and hair. It is the channels and network vessels (*i.e.*, smaller connecting vessels) which connect the inside and the outside of the body. It is through these channels and network vessels that the viscera and bowels connect with their corresponding body tissues.

The channels and network vessel system is a unique feature of traditional Chinese medicine. These channels and vessels are different from the circulatory, nervous, or lymphatic systems. The earliest reference to these channels and vessels is in *Nei Jing (Inner Classic)*, a text written around the 2nd or 3rd century BCE.

The channels and vessels perform two basic functions. They are the pathways by which the qi and blood circulate through the body and between the organs and tissues. Additionally, as mentioned above, the channels connect the viscera and bowels internally with the exterior part of the body. This channel and vessel system functions in the body much like the world information communication network. The channels allow the various parts of our body to cooperate and interact to maintain our lives.

This channel and network vessel system is complex. There are 12 primary channels, 6 yin and 6 yang, each with a specific pathway through the external body and connected with an internal organ (see diagram below). There are also extraordinary vessels, sinew channels, channel divergences, main network vessels, and

29

ultimately countless finer and finer network vessels permeating the entire body. All of these form a closed loop or circuit similar to but distinct from the Western circulatory system.

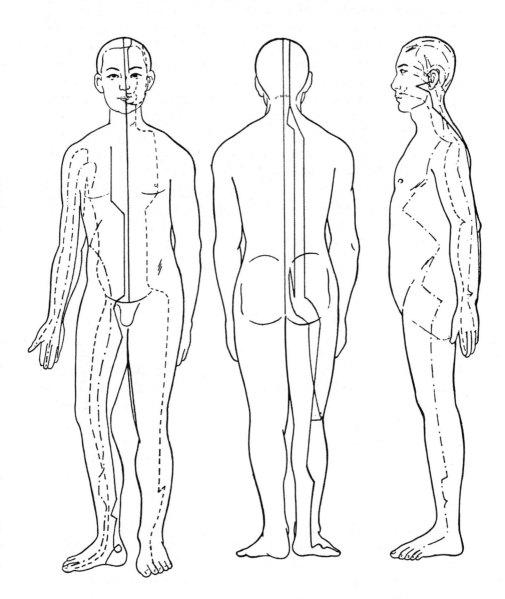

Acupuncture points are places located on the major channels where there is a special concentration of qi and blood. Because of the relatively more qi and blood accumulated at these places, the sites act as switches which can potentially control the flow of qi and blood in the channel on which the point is located. By stimulating these points in any of a number of different ways, one can speed up or slow down, make more or reduce, warm or cool down the qi and blood flowing in the channels and vessels. The main ways of stimulating these points and thus adjusting the flow of qi and blood in the channels and vessels is to needle them and to heat them by moxibustion.[11] Other commonly used ways of stimulating these points and thus adjusting the qi and blood flowing through the channels and vessels are massage, cupping, the application of magnets, and the application of various herbal medicinals. If the channels and vessels are the pathways over which the qi and blood flow, then the acupuncture points are the places where this flow can be adjusted.

---

[11] Moxibustion refers to adding heat to an acupuncture point or area of the body by burning a dried herb, Folium Artemisae Argyii (*Ai Ye*), Oriental mugwort, on, over, or near the area to be warmed.

The Menstrual Cycle in Chinese Medicine

I t is said in Chinese medicine that men and women are basically the same. However, women have a uterus and thus they menstruate, can conceive, give birth, and lactate. The menses themselves are a discharge of blood. For this discharge to take place, two things have to occur. First, a superabundance of blood must accumulate in the uterus for it to eventually spill over as the menstruate. And secondly, the qi and blood must be freely and uninhibitedly flowing in order to allow this brimming over. This means that, in order to understand menstruation, one must understand how blood is created and what might affect the free and uninhibited flow of qi and blood.

The creation of blood

There are three viscera which participate in the creation of the blood. These are the kidneys, spleen, and heart. The heart is the place where the blood is "turned red" or finally created. However, first the spleen must send up the finest essence of food and liquids extracted in the process of digestion. If the spleen does not send up this finest essence of food and liquids there will be insufficient supplies for the heart to transform these into blood. In addition, the kidneys must send up some essence to also participate in the creation of blood. One can think of this as somewhat similar to adding some sourdough starter in order to make a new batch of sourdough bread.

In other words, if the kidney lacks sufficient essence, if the spleen fails to digest the finest essence of food and liquids and send this upward, and if the heart, for any reason, cannot fulfill its function of "turning the blood red," then there may be insufficient creation of blood. In addition, it is the heart's job to spread the blood to the rest of the body and eventually move it down to the uterus. It is said in Chinese medicine that first the blood goes to nourish and moisten the viscera and bowels. Then it goes into the channels and vessels. From there it nourishes and moistens the rest of the tissues of the body, and what collects in the uterus is what is left over after the blood has performed all these other jobs. When enough blood collects in the uterus to fill it, it overflows as the menses. Typically, a young to middle-aged, healthy woman will produce such a superabundance accumulating in the uterus once every 28-30 days.

The control of the blood

Although normal menstruation cannot occur if there is insufficient blood accumulated in the uterus, it can occur either too early or too late if the flow of blood is not controlled properly. Just as there are three viscera which engender and transform the blood, there are three viscera which govern or control the blood. These are the heart, liver, and spleen. It is said that the heart qi governs the blood. Above we have seen that this means that it is the heart qi which "stirs" or pushes the blood. If the heart qi does not move the blood, the blood cannot move on its own. Thus it is said:

If the qi moves, the blood moves. If the qi stops, the blood stops.

In actual fact, the heart gets its qi primarily from the spleen. So a sufficiency of spleen qi is necessary for there to be enough heart qi to move the blood. In addition, the spleen qi restrains and contains the blood within its channels and vessels. If the spleen qi is too weak, it may allow the blood to seep out prematurely or it may not cut off menstruation when it should. And finally, the liver stores the blood. It is the liver's job to regulate the amount of blood in circulation. It is the liver qi which performs this function. If the liver qi spreads freely, then the blood moves. If the liver qi becomes depressed and stagnant, then the blood will also eventually become depressed and static.

One may find it hard at first to distinguish the difference between the spleen and the liver's role in maintaining the free and uninhibited flow of blood. It is the spleen qi ultimately (via the heart) which provides the motivating force behind the propulsion of the blood. It is the liver which allows the blood to flow freely through its channels and vessels. If, for instance, one has gas in their car and the car is in good working order, one may have the power to move one's car. However, if one is stopped at a red light, one may not have the permission to move the car even though the power is there. In terms of the heart, spleen and liver, the flow of blood is the same. The heart and spleen provide the motivating power, but it is the liver qi which allows that blood to flow freely or not.

If, for any reason, one of these three viscera does not function correctly in terms of the flow of blood, this may impede the free and timely flow of the menstruate.

The four phases of the menstrual cycle

Chinese gynecologists divide the menstrual cycle into four, roughly seven day periods. Phase one begins the day the menses end. If one counts the days of the menstrual cycle from the first day of the onset of menstruation, this means that phase one typically begins on day four, five, six, or seven. The uterus had discharged its accumulated blood and this leaves the body relatively empty or vacuous of blood. Because blood is created, at least in part out of kidney essence and because, compared to yang qi, essence is a type of yin substance, during phase one, the body busies itself with making more yin and blood to replenish that which was discharged. Therefore, in Chinese gynecology, we say that phase one corresponds to yin and the emphasis in the body is on replenishing yin blood.

35

Phase two correponds to the days surrounding ovulation. Up till now, the body has been replenishing its yin. However, for ovulation to occur, yin must transform into yang. This transformation of yin into yang corresponds to the rise in basal body temperature which occurs after ovulation.[12] If there is insufficient yin, it cannot transform into yang. Conversely, if there is insufficient yang, it cannot trasnform yin. In addition, if either the qi and blood are not flowing freely, this transformation may also be impeded. Generally, phase two corresponds to days 10-16 in the monthly cycle and it corresponds to yang in the same way that phase one corresponds to yin.

Phase three corresponds to the premenstruum and to the qi. For things to go as they should in the woman's body, yang qi must stay strong enough long enough and the qi must flow freely and in the right directions. Many of the signs and symptoms of PMS have to do with the yang qi not being strong enough or the qi (and therefore the blood) not flowing freely. Phase three may be counted from day 17 to the day before menstruation, i.e., day 28, and corresponds to qi.

Phase four is the menstruation itself. Since the onset of menstruation is counted as day one in the cycle, phase four may last anywhere from one or two days to six or seven depending on the individual woman's constitution and age. Because menstruation is a downward discharge of blood according to Chinese medicine, phase four corresponds to the blood.

When looked at from this perspective, the menstrual cycle is made up of four (not always equal) segments corresponding to yin, yang, qi and blood. This relationship is shown in the chart below.

---

[12] Basal body temperature refers to one's resting temperature when taken the first thing upon waking in the morning before getting up, dressing, eating, or doing anything else. It is analogous to one's resting pulse or one's basal metabolic rate. Plotting one's basal body temperature on a graph is one way of determining if and when a woman is ovulating.

Qi, Blood, Yin & Yang
vis-a-vis Menstrual Cycle

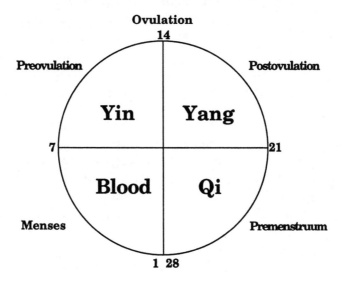

Problems may occur in any of these four phases and may occur for reasons other than the dominant correspondence in that phase. However, when a problem occurs in any of these four phases, the Chinese doctor will first investigate to see if the dominant correspondence, whether yin, yang, qi, or blood, is behaving as it should at that time. Since PMS occurs in the premenstruum or phase three, most premenstrual complaints are attributed, either directly or indirectly, to problems with the flow of qi.

Age and the menstrual cycle

In Chinese medicine, the doctor takes everything about the patient into account. This includes their bodily constitution, their temperament, their lifestyle and occupation, and their age. There is a famous saying in Chinese gynecology which runs:

37

In adolescent (girls), blame the kidneys.
In middle-aged (women), blame the liver.
In older (women), blame the spleen.

When adolescent girls first begin menstruating, their cycles are often irregular. They may go several months or more between menses and their periods may not come regularly every 28-30 days until several years after menarche or the beginning of menstruation. In Chinese medicine, this is explained as being due to the immaturity of the kidneys. Because the kidneys must supply essence to create the superabundance of blood necessary for menstruation to occur naturally, if the kidneys are not mature, they may not supply the needed essence every 28 days. Because maturation is not an all or nothing affair, as every parent knows, the amount of essence and, therefore, the regularity of the menstrual cycle may fluctuate for some time before it becomes stable. So it is said, "In adolescent (girls), blame the kidneys."

Once the kidneys have become stable and mature and menstruation occurs on a regular basis, then most gynecological diseases are impugned to the liver. In Chinese medicine, the liver is called the "tempermental viscus." This means that it is easily damaged or upset by emotional influences. In particular, it is said that, "The liver likes orderly reaching." This means that the liver qi likes to spread out without restriction or hindrance like a large broad–leafed tree. When the liver encounters frustration, its coursing and discharging of the qi is inhibited. The qi cannot flow as freely as it wants and it becomes depressed and stagnant. The qi becomes bottled up, and this gives rise to anger and irritability since anger is the emotion associated with Chinese liver dis-ease.

However, when the qi becomes depressed and stuck, this also affects the flow of blood and body fluids, since it is the qi which moves and transforms both of these. Menstruation is the discharge of blood, and this discharge requires the free flow of qi to occur normally. Therefore, if the qi becomes depressed, the blood does not move, and if the blood does not move, menstruation cannot occur normally.

It is a fact of life that adults cannot do everything they want to do at the moment we want to do it. Learning to delay gratification is one of the things all adults learn, whether we like it or not. However, when we cannot do what we want to do when we want to do it, this affects our liver's coursing and discharging and the free spreading of our qi. Hence, it is a rare adult who has so few thwarted desires that their qi and blood flows absolutely freely and uninhibitedly. In actual clinical fact, almost all adults have some manifestations of liver depression qi stagnation, and in women, this almost always causes some menstrual irregularity. Therefore, because a certain level of liver depression qi stagnation is endemic in being an adult (at least in a civilized society where one must practice certain restraints), it is said, "In middle-aged (women), blame the liver."

According to the *Nei Jing (The Inner Classic)*, the "bible of Chinese medicine" compiled sometime in the second or third century BCE, the spleen and stomach begin to decline at around 35 years of age. Because the spleen and its helper the stomach are the source of the creation of qi and blood out of the food and liquids we eat, this decline in spleen-stomach function corresponds to a decline in the amounts of qi and blood produced. Therefore, from approximately 35 years of age till menopause, the spleen must struggle to produce enough qi and blood to nourish and empower the entire body and create a surplus of blood to flow over as the menstruate. This puts a heavy burden on the spleen and causes many women to show pronounced or more pronounced signs and symptoms of spleen weakness after the mid-30s and through the 40s. In such cases, the liver depression qi stagnation does not automatically go away. In fact, as we will see below, it may even get worse. However, when it comes to emphasis, this liver depression qi stagnation may not produce as many signs and symptoms as the spleen vacuity or weakness. Thus it is said, "In older (women), blame the spleen."[13]

As we will see in the next chapter, there is no PMS without liver depression qi stagnation. However, as a woman moves into her mid-30s and through her 40s, PMS is not just due to the liver but also due to the spleen and the other viscera and bowels associated with the spleen and liver, most notably the heart and kidneys. Therefore, age plays its part in understanding the Chinese cause and treatment of PMS and why it often gets worse, not better, in women as they age.

Menopause and Chinese medicine

Eventually, the body in its wisdom recognizes it is not healthy to try to create qi and blood to nourish and empower the rest of the body at the same time as continuing to menstruate regularly with the loss of blood that that necessarily entails. Therefore, the body initiates a transformation which, from the Chinese medical point of view, is literally a "change in life." The Chinese medical literature does not say exactly how, but at some point, the heart ceases sending blood down to collect in the uterus. Just as maturation does not happen all at once, this process is also a gradual one in most women. Therefore, the menses do not just suddenly cease, but menopause is commonly preceded by months or even years of a certain amount of menstrual irregularity. Nevertheless, sooner or later, the heart stops sending blood down to the uterus. Instead, the kidneys are now free to send essence up

---

[13] Obviously, 35 years of age or even 45 years of age is not considered old nowadays. The reader should keep in mind, however, that in ancient China when this saying was coined, due to hard physical labor, repeated and excessive pregnancies, and periodic famines and pestilences, many women were aged by their mid to late forties. In any case, these ages are not meant as absolutes but rather as a continuum, with spleen weakness becoming an important part of many women's Chinese medical diagnosis after approximately 35 years of age.

to accumulate in the heart where it joins with the qi and blood sent up by the spleen and becomes spirit.

Thus the woman goes from mother of babies to mother of her tribe, the *sage femme* or wise woman full of spirit. If this change occurs smoothly, it naturally puts an end to any PMS, since there is no menses let alone a pre-menses. Unfortunately, the smooth cessation of menstruation is, like all other transformations in the body, dependent on the free flow of liver qi. Since there is no PMS without liver depression qi stagnation,[14] women's menopausal complaints tend to be, both in Chinese theory and my own clinical experience, proportional to the severity of their PMS. In other words, PMS and menopausal syndrome are ultimately not two separate diseases but an unfortunate continuum whose core issue is liver depression qi stagnation. Although we will discuss this slide from PMS into menopausal complaints somewhat below, readers interested in learning more about Chinese medicine and menopause should see Honora Lee Wolfe's *Menopause, A Second Spring: Making a Smooth Transition with Chinese Medicine* also published by Blue Poppy Press.

---

[14] Liver depression qi stagnation is the proper name of a pathological pattern in Chinese medicine. It is often abbreviated to either just liver depression or qi stagnation, or it may be referred to simply as liver qi. When speaking of the other four viscera or the bowels, if one says heart qi or spleen qi, one is referring to the healthy qi of that organ. But because the liver qi is so often depressed and stagnant in adults, this is the only case where simply saying liver qi almost always refers to a pathological condition of depression and stagnation.

The Chinese Mechanisms of PMS

Although Chinese doctors have been treating premenstrual complaints for centuries if not millenia, PMS is a relatively recent addition to the Chinese medical literature. In Chinese, premenstrual syndrome is frequently translated as *jing xing xian qi zhu zheng*. *Jing xing* means menstrual movement. *Xian qi* means before the period. And *zhu zheng* means various pathological conditions or syndrome. This is a modern Chinese attempt to literally translate PMS into Chinese. This new category is now beginning to show up in Chinese gynecology texts and articles. However, if one looks, for instance, at the table of contents of the gynecology section of the *Yi Zong Jin Jian (The Golden Mirror of Ancestral Medicine)*—the famous Qing dynasty compendium of medicine published in 1749 CE—under the subheading of regulating menstruation, one finds a group of conditions each prefixed by the words *jing xing*. These words mean menstrual movement. The implication in Chinese is that these conditions all in some way have to do with pathological mechanisms occurring when the menstrual blood is moving to and out of the uterus. Thus, in the older Chinese medical literature, these *jing xing* diseases refer to what we now group as the various conditions constituting premenstrual syndrome.

The list of such menstrual movement conditions is open-ended. Some Chinese gynecology texts only give one or two menstrual movement diseases, while others give dozens. In fact, we can say that any complaint or pathological condition occurring during the premenstruum or the menses themselves (including the 150 PMS symptoms recognized by Western medicine) can be prefixed with the words menstrual movement. Therefore, there are some commonly seen menstrual movement diseases and there are some pretty unusual ones. When I teach professional practitioners how to diagnose and treat PMS, I ask the women in the audience to name the various complaints they know either from their own or their patients' experience to be possible premenstrually. Below is a sample of such a list:

Irritability
Easy crying
Impaired memory
Lack of concentration
Lack of clear thinking
Fatigue
Loss of coordination
Swollen, tender breasts
Growth of cystic lumps in
    the breast
Edema of the face, hands,
    and feet
Lower abdominal distention
Lower abdominal cramping
Lack of strength
Headaches, including
    migraines
Catching a cold or flu
Cravings for sweets
Cravings for salt
Cravings for carbohydrates
Increased appetite in
    general

Lack of appetite
Insomnia
Night sweats
Low back pain
Acne
Hives
Vaginitis and vaginal sores
Heart palpitations
Diarrhea
Nausea and vomiting
Constipation
Flatulence
Painful and/or frequent
    urination
Loss of libido
Spotting of blood
Nosebleed
Coughing or vomiting blood
Blood in the urine or stools
Worsening of eczema or
    psoriasis
Cold sores

Any of these complaints can and do occur cyclically during the premenstruum in some women. When they occur on a regular basis before each menstruation, they are prefaced by the words "menstrual movement", as in menstrual movement diarrhea or menstrual movement hives. Most women with PMS will have several of these complaints. It is the fact that PMS does include more than a single complaint or symptom that it is called a syndrome, remembering that in Chinese, syndrome is translated as "various conditions."

Therefore, potentially any abnormal discomfort or complaint, sign or symptom can be labelled as PMS in Chinese medicine, not just the main ones mentioned in *The Merck Manual* above. More unusual complaints discussed in the Chinese medical literature include menstrual movement pneumothorax and menstrual movement lip swelling and pain. The only criterion for a complaint to be labelled as a menstrual movement disease in Chinese medicine is that it must occur on a regular basis before or during the menses.

This means that PMS in modern Chinese gynecology is actually no one thing. The actual complaints that any given patient may present are highly variable and idiosyncratic. Nonetheless, it is my clinical experience that Chinese medicine can diagnose and successfully treat every possible premenstrual complaint any woman can present.

That being said, let me first discuss the common textbook patterns associated with PMS in the contemporary Chinese gynecology textbook literature. Both Sun Jiu-ling, author of *Fu Ke Zheng Zhi (Gynecological Patterns & Treatments)*, and Zhu Cheng-han, author of *Zhong Yi Fu Ke (Chinese Medical Gynecology)*, list PMS as a disease category similar to modern Western medicine. Sun discusses three patterns in the TCM treatment of PMS. To these same three, Zhu adds a fourth. Understanding these four basic patterns will enable the practitioner to understand the mechanisms behind most of the various signs and symptoms associated with PMS. However, after discussing these four patterns, I will add several more in order to give a more complete picture.

Disease causes, disease mechanisms

The root cause of PMS is almost always a disharmony between the liver and spleen. Due to emotional stress and frustration, the liver becomes depressed and the qi becomes stagnant. Due to worry, lack of exercise, overfatigue, or improper diet, the spleen may become vacuous and weak. Because, in Chinese medicine, it is said that the liver controls the spleen, if the liver becomes depressed, this can cause or worsen spleen vacuity or weakness. Conversely, if the spleen is vacuous and weak, this may allow the liver to become or become even more depressed. Liver depression tends to worsen or arise during the premenstruum because the blood that was nourishing, softening, and harmonizing the liver is now being sent down to nourish the uterus. If there is not sufficient blood for both these purposes, the liver may not receive sufficient nourishment so that it can perform its duty of controlling the coursing and discharge, *i.e.*, the free flow, of the qi. If the liver does not course and discharge, the qi does not move freely and becomes stagnant.

It is the spleen which is the root of qi and blood engenderment and transformation. If the spleen is vacuous and weak, then it may not engender and transform qi and blood sufficiently. If the spleen does not engender blood sufficiently, then, as we have just seen above, liver blood may become insufficient to allow the liver to perform its function of coursing and discharging the qi. On the other hand, if the spleen does not engender the qi sufficiently, the qi will lack its motivating force to move. Thus it is easy to see how closely these two viscera are related in terms of the free flow of the qi. The liver allows the qi to flow freely, but it is the spleen which is the ultimate source of the qi's power to move. Hence liver depression and spleen vacuity typically go hand in hand in clinical practice. In addition, we should remember that, because of their monthly loss of blood, women's spleens must work harder at producing blood then men's spleens must. This also predisposes women in particular towards a spleen insufficiency. In my experience, liver depression-spleen vacuity weakness is usually the root mechanism behind PMS. I have never seen a single case of PMS in 17 years of clinical practice without at least some element of liver depression.

According to Chinese medical theory, if the liver becomes depressed and qi stagnant, this may eventually transform into pathological heat. Remember that the qi is inherently warm. If the qi becomes stuck and accumulates, backing up under pressure, all this depressed and stagnant yang qi will transform into what is called transformative or depressive heat. Over time, this pathological heat, being by nature yang, will consume and dry out kidney yin. Since, in Chinese medicine, yin is supposed to control yang, if kidney yin becomes vacuous and weak, liver yang may become hyperactive. Since fire burns upward and the heart and lungs are located above the liver, this pathological heat may also accumulate in the heart and/or lungs, disturbing either or both heart and lung function.

As mentioned above, since the spleen is the root of the engenderment and transformation of blood, if the spleen becomes weak, the blood may also become vacuous. Since some essence from the kidneys is required in order to make new blood, it is said in Chinese medicine that blood and essence share a common source. What this means in terms of disease mechanisms is that enduring blood vacuity may lead to insufficiency of kidney essence. This may aggravate any tendency to kidney yin vacuity already caused by damage due to enduring heat.

Because the spleen is also in charge of moving and transforming liquids, if the spleen becomes weak, water dampness may accumulate. Dampness which is yin, being thick and turbid, may further block the free flow of qi which is yang, thus aggravating liver depression. Dampness may also congeal and transform into phlegm. This phlegm even further impedes the free flow of qi and may lodge between the skin and flesh, in the channels and network vessels, and in what are known as the clear orifices of the heart and head. Phlegm blocking the clear orifices of the heart

47

gives rise to mental emotional problems. The clear orifices of the head refer to the sensory organs of the eyes, ears, nose, and mouth. If phlegm blocks any of these, then there will be some disturbance in the function of the associated sense. For instance, if the orifices of the eyes are blocked by phlegm, then there will be vision problems. If the orifices of the ears are blocked, there will be hearing problems, etc.

In Chinese medicine, the functioning of the spleen and stomach are likened to a pot on a stove and the process of digestion and the production of qi and blood is likened to the cooking of sour mash and distillation of alcohol. According to this metaphor, qi and blood are the distillation of foods and liquids cooked and transformed by the spleen and stomach. However, the ultimate source of heat for the spleen and stomach to do their job is the kidney fire or kidney yang. This kidney fire can be likened to the pilot light in a stove. If it goes out, the burners cannot function. Therefore, if the spleen remains chronically weak, since kidney yang is the source of the heat of the middle burner, *i.e.,* the spleen and stomach, kidney yang may also become weak. Since kidney essence is the material basis of both kidney yin and yang, this process can be accelerated if there is long-term blood vacuity. On the other hand, enduring kidney yang vacuity and weakness will also impair blood production as well.

All this may seem pretty complicated to the novice in Chinese medicine. As I said at the beginning of this book, Chinese medicine is a very complex system of thought. Even if one cannot grasp the meanings and implications of all of the above on their first reading, the reader should by now agree that Chinese medicine is by no means a primitive folk medicine. As we will see below, there are even a few more mechanisms which may occur as ramifications of these main disease mechanisms. However, the above mechanisms are the root of most premenstrual signs and symptoms. If one understands these mechanisms and has a sound grasp of the basic theories of Chinese medicine discussed above, one can figure out *a rational explanation for any sign or symptom any woman may experience before her menses.*

Treatment according to pattern discrimination

The hallmark of professional Chinese medicine is what is known as "treatment based on pattern discrimination." Modern Western medicine bases its treatment on a disease diagnosis. This means that two patients diagnosed as suffering from the same disease will get the same treatment. Traditional Chinese medicine also takes the patient's disease diagnosis into account. However, the choice of treatment is not based on the disease so much as it is on what is called the patient's pattern, and it is treatment based on pattern discrimination which is what makes Chinese medicine the holistic, safe, and effective medicine it is.

In order to explain the difference between a disease and pattern, let us take headache for example. Everyone who is diagnosed as suffering from a headache has to, by definition, have some pain in their head. In modern Western medicine and other medical systems which primarily prescribe on the basis of a disease diagnosis, one can talk about "headache medicines." However, amongst headache sufferers, one may be a man and the other a woman. One may be old and the other young. One may be fat and the other skinny. One may have pain on the right side of her head and the other may have pain on the left. In one case, the pain may be throbbing and continuous, while the other person's pain may be very sharp but intermittent. In one case, they may also have indigestion, a tendency to loose stools, lack of warmth in their feet, red eyes, a dry mouth and desire for cold drinks, while the other person has a wet, weeping, crusty skin rash with red borders, a tendency to hay fever, ringing in their ears, and dizziness when they stand up. In Chinese medicine just as in modern Western medicine, both these patients suffer from headache. That is their disease diagnosis. However, they also suffer from a whole host of other complaints, have very different types of headaches, and very different constitutions, ages, and sex.

In Chinese medicine, the patient's pattern is made up from all these other signs and symptoms and other information. Thus, in Chinese medicine, the pattern describes *the totality of the person as a unique individual*. And in Chinese medicine, treatment is designed to rebalance that entire pattern of imbalance as well as address the major complaint or disease. Thus, there is a saying in Chinese medicine:

> One disease, different treatments
> Different diseases, same treatment

This means that, in Chinese medicine, two patients with the same named disease diagnosis may receive different treatments *if their Chinese medical patterns are different*, while two patients diagnosed with different named diseases may receive the same treatment *if their Chinese medical pattern is the same*. In other words, in Chinese medicine, treatment is predicated primarily on one's pattern discrimination, not on one's named disease diagnosis. Therefore, each person is treated individually. There is no PMS formula or PMS herb. Nor is there any magic PMS acupuncture point.

Since every patient gets just the treatment which is right to restore balance to their particular body, there are also no unwanted side effects. Side effects come from forcing one part of the body to behave while causing an imbalance in some other part. The medicine may have fit part of the problem but not the entirety of the patient as an individual. This is like robbing Peter to pay Paul. Since Chinese medicine sees the entire body (and mind!) as a single, unified whole, curing imbalance in one area of the body while causing it in another is unacceptable.

Below is a description of the major Chinese medical patterns at work in PMS:

Liver depression qi stagnation

Main symptoms: Premenstrual breast distention and pain, chest and side of the rib pain, lower abdominal distention and pain, discomfort in the stomach and epigastrium, diminished appetite, possible delayed menstruation whose amount is either scanty or profuse, clots within the menstrual blood, menses unable to come easily, a normal or slightly dark tongue with thin, white fur, and a bowstring,[15] fine pulse

Treatment principles: Course the liver and move the qi, rectify the blood and regulate the menses

Spleen-kidney yang vacuity

Main symptoms: Edema either before or after the menses, dizziness, lumbar soreness and weary extremities, reduced appetite, loose stools or diarrhea before the menses, stomach and epigastric distention and fullness, lack of warmth in the hands and feet, a pale facial complexion, menses scanty in amount, a fat tongue with thin, white or slimy, white fur, and a deep, fine, weak pulse

In actual clinical fact, this pattern never presents in this simple, discreet manner in PMS. But spleen qi and kidney yang vacuity do typically complicate most women's PMS in their late 30s and 40s. According to my clinical experience, there will also be liver depression as well in all cases. Therefore, in clinical practice, one chooses a prescription which remedies spleen vacuity if that is more pronounced and then modifies that for liver depression, while, if liver depression is the dominant pattern, then one

---

[15] There are 28 main pulse types in Chinese medicine, the bowstring pulse being one of these. It feels like its name implies—like a taut violin or bowstring. It is almost universally felt in women with PMS.

chooses a formula for liver depression and modifies that for spleen and kidney vacuity.

Treatment principles: Warm the kidneys, fortify the the spleen, and disinhibit water

Heart-spleen dual vacuity

Main symptoms: Heart palpitations either before or after the menses, loss of sleep, lassitude of the spirit, lack of strength, face slightly puffy, amount of menses either profuse or scanty but pale in color, a pale tongue with thin, white fur, and a soggy, small or fine, weak pulse

Heart-spleen dual vacuity means heart blood vacuity and spleen qi vacuity. If heart blood is more vacuous, the amount of the menstruate is scanty. If spleen qi vacuity is more prominent, the amount of discharge is profuse. However, in both cases, the color of the menstruate tends to be pale. Likewise, if the spleen is vacuous and, therefore, also damp, the pulse will be soggy.[16] But if blood is vacuous, the pulse will be fine. As with the above pattern, this one also is rarely if ever seen in its simple, discreet form in clinical practice. Commonly, if there is heart blood vacuity, this merely complicates liver depression and spleen vacuity. If the liver depression is secondary in importance, then one would choose a guiding formula which primarily supplements and nourishes the heart and spleen, modifying it for liver depression. If liver depression is primary, then one would modify a formula from under that pattern.

Treatment principles: Supplement and nourish heart and spleen qi and blood

---

[16] A soggy pulse is another of the main 28 pulse images of Chinese medicine. It refers to a pulse which is floating, fine, and forceless.

Kidney vacuity, liver effulgence

Main symptoms: Menstruation either early or late, lumbar soreness, numb extremities, one-sided headache, tinnitus, blurred vision, distention and pain feels as if it stretches from the lower abdomen to the chest and breasts, frequent, short urination, length of menstruation short and amount profuse, tongue fur shiny and peeled with a fat tongue and purple edges, and a deep, small, bowstring pulse

Although not stated in the Chinese title of this pattern, liver qi depression and stagnation are a part of this scenario. This is evidenced by the feeling of lower abdominal distention and pain reaching to the chest and breasts and also by the bowstring pulse. In this case, liver depression transforms into fire and causes the blood to move recklessly. Therefore, the amount of menses is profuse. But because liver blood is relatively vacuous or empty, the length of the menses is short.

Treatment principles: Boost the kidneys and regulate the liver

The real deal

Although textbook discriminations such as the one above make it seem like all the practitioner has to do is match up their patient's symptoms with one of the afore mentioned patterns and then prescribe the recommended guiding formula, in actual clinical practice, one usually encounters combinations of the above discreet patterns and their related disease mechanisms or progressions. In trying to identify all the mechanisms I have encountered in women with PMS, I have come up with a list of 20.

These are:

Liver depression qi stagnation
Depressive heat
Spleen qi vacuity
Spleen dampness
Liver blood vacuity
Kidney yin vacuity
Spleen-kidney yang vacuity
Replete heat in the heart,
    lungs, and/or stomach
Vacuity heat in the heart,
    lungs, and/or stomach
Heart qi and/or blood vacuity
Liver yang hyperactivity

Liver fire flaring above
Stirring of liver wind
Food stagnation
Phlegm confounding the
    orifices
Phlegm fire
Damp heat accumulating
    below
Blood stasis
External invasion
Retained evils or deep-lying
    warm evils

In all cases of PMS, liver qi plays a central role. This is because, the premenstruum and the menstrual movement are about yang reaching its maximum and transforming into yin just as ovulation is about yin reaching its maximum and transforming into yang. Such transformation can only proceed freely and correctly if the qi mechanism is free-flowing and uninhibited. The qi mechanism's free and uninhibited flow is dependent on the liver's coursing and discharge. Therefore, liver depression and qi stagnation are at the heart of every woman's PMS. No matter what other disease mechanisms are at work, the presence and degree of premenstrual complaints are directly proportional to the presence of liver qi.

However, because of the interrelationships between the liver and all the other viscera and bowels of Chinese medicine and between the qi, blood, fluids, and essence, liver depression qi stagnation may be complicated or evolve into a number of other patterns. Therefore, in clinical practice, one must identify the main disease mechanism currently at work and choose a guiding formula or treatment based on rebalancing that imbalance. Then this guiding formula is modified to address all of the patient's associated disease mechanisms and signs and symptoms. However, if a mechanism or symptom will disappear by merely rebalancing some more fundamental mechanism, such secondary or dependent mechanisms and symptoms need not be addressed specifically.

If one understands the interrelationships between the above 20 mechanisms, they can then diagnose and understand *any* premenstrual symptom of *any* woman. These 20 mechanisms or patterns are not just a random collection of patterns. There is an underlying logic to this list.

We have already discussed the relationships between the first seven mechanisms above. If liver depression transforms into depressive heat, that heat may counterflow upward and harass the heart, lungs, and/or stomach. On the other hand, if liver blood-kidney vacuity gives rise to vacuity heat, this vacuity heat may also counterflow upward to harass the heart, lungs, and/or stomach and damage their yin fluids. Because both heart qi and blood have their source in the spleen's engenderment and transformation of water and grains, if the spleen is vacuous and weak, this may easily give rise to either heart blood or heart qi vacuity. If depressive heat damages yin, yang will become effulgent and give rise to liver yang hyperactivity. If such liver yang hyperactivity becomes even worse, it may become liver fire flaring above, while liver fire and/or liver blood vacuity may engender internal stirring of liver wind.

In the Yuan dynasty (1280-168 CE), Zhu Dan-xi, one of the four great masters of medicine of his time, explained that, if qi becomes stagnant and the spleen becomes weak, food stagnation is easily engendered. Food stagnation means food which sits in the stomach undigested. Such food stagnation may also transform depressive heat. If dampness due to the spleen not moving and transporting fluids gathers and endures, it may congeal into phlegm. However, phlegm may also be due to intense heat steaming and fuming the fluids, congealing them into phlegm like cooking pudding on a stove top. In either case, phlegm, being a yin depression, obstructs the free and uninhibited flow of qi and blood. It may gather and obstruct in the area between the skin and muscles or flesh, within the viscera and bowels, and within the channels and network vessels. It may also confound and block the clear orifices, *i.e.*, the sensory organs of the head, or the orifices of the heart. If the clear orifices are blocked, there will be diminished or loss of sensual acuity of the associated orifice. If the orifices of the heart are confounded, there will be disturbed or diminished mental-emotional function.

However, dampness, being heavy and turbid, tends to precolate and pour downward. Because it too is a yin depression, it obstructs the free flow of qi, blood, and fluids. If damp depression gives rise to depressive heat, then dampness may become damp heat. It is also possible for liver depression-transformative heat to stew the juices and give rise to damp heat. If qi stagnation fails to move the blood, the blood will stop and become static. Thus, if liver depression is bad enough or lasts long enough, it may give rise to blood stasis. Static blood is like silt in the blood vessels, and like silt in a river or canal, it may eventually clog and obstruct the flow of blood in the affected area. Blood stasis is mainly associated with pain, such as menstrual or premenstrual lower abdominal pain, premenstrual breast pain, headache, or other relatively severe aches and pains which are fixed in location and tend to be sharp or piercing in nature.

Because the spleen and stomach are the source of the defensive qi, if the spleen becomes vacuous and weak premenstrually, there may be a defensive qi vacuity. Such a defensive qi vacuity premenstrually is often aggravated by blood vacuity. Because the blood is sent down to the uterus before menstruation, this leaves the upper body relatively empty and insufficient of blood in women whose blood production tends to be poor. The blood and the constructive qi are closely related. Therefore, such a blood and constructive qi vacuity in the upper body leads to a disharmony between the defensive and constructive qi which easily allows for external pathogens to take advantage of this vacuity and enter. This then results in recurrent colds or flus before the menses.

56

It is also possible that either "retained evils" or "deep-lying warm evils" may become active during the premenstruum. Retained evils are pathogens that have invaded the body at some previous time. Due to lack of or erroneous treatment, these pathogens have not all been eliminated from the body at the time of their invasion and subsequent disease. If some of these pathogens linger, they may be relatively latent. However, given the proper internal environment, they may become active again. Hidden or deep-lying warm evils are warm or damp heat pathogens which enter the body but do not cause disease at that time. Rather, they lie latent until the internal environment is conducive to their exuberance and activity. Because dampness tends to accumulate premenstrually and because there is often depressive heat premenstrually at the same time as there is a righteous qi vacuity affecting the spleen and/or kidneys, either retained or deep-lying warm evils often find the premenstruum a time when the internal environment is conducive to their exuberance and activity. The Chinese theories about retained and deep-lying evils helps explain premenstrual outbreaks of herpes and cold sores.

All signs and symptoms of PMS can be diagnosed and treated according to Chinese medicine based on various combinations of the above disease mechanisms and patterns. In order to make this work, one must have a firm grasp of the defining or main symptoms of each pattern. Such a grasp is normally beyond most laypersons. Therefore, to get the full benefits of Chinese medicine, it is best if one receives a pattern discrimination from a qualified professional practitioner. Below I will discuss how and where to find such practitioners in the United States. However, there is a lot one can do on one's own if one has only a general idea of their Chinese medical pattern. Hopefully, readers with PMS have identified some of their own signs and symptoms from under the patterns discussed above. If so, see which pattern includes the majority of your signs and symptoms. Then write that down. It is probable that that is the main pattern or disease mechanism accounting for your PMS. Even if you only address the main pattern and miss some of the minor complications, you should experience some relief of your symptoms. And remember, every woman with PMS does have liver depression qi stagnation either as her main pattern or a secondary mechanism. So following the dietary, exercise, and lifestyle recommendations for that pattern are universally helpful.

How This System Works in Real-life

Using all the above information on the theory of Chinese medicine and the patterns and their mechanisms of the main PMS complaints discussed in the Chinese medical literature, one can diagnose and, therefore, treat any premenstrual complaint or combination of complaints with Chinese medicine.

Denise's case

Take Denise, for instance, whom I introduced at the beginning of this book. Each month she is irritable and upset before her period. Not only does she get angry for little or no reason, but she tends to cry at the drop of a hat. In addition, her periods tend to be late, coming anywhere between 33-45 days apart. Before her menses start, she has lower abdominal bloating and cramping for a couple of days. During the first few hours of her period, she has more severe cramps which are relieved by rubbing, applying heat, or, if she can get herself to do it, some light exercise. In addition, her breasts become sore and distended before her menses with her nipples becoming especially sensitive and sore or inflamed feeling. Denise tends to be constipated right up until the day her menses start, and then she has loose stools for a day. Part of the reason Denise gets irritable premenstrually is that she feels more fatigued at that time. If she eats a large meal, her abdomen becomes bloated and it feels like her food is just sitting in her stomach all day. Nevertheless, she finds that her appetite is increased premenstrually, especially craving sweets and carbohydrates. To add insult to injury, a few days before her period, Denise gets two or three pimples at the corners of her mouth.

These are fairly large and red. Her tongue is a normal color with slightly yellow fur. However, her tongue is a little swollen, and one can see the indentations of her teeth along its edges. There is a bitter taste in her mouth when Denise wakes up in the morning. Her pulse is bowstring overall. However, her right pulse in the position which corresponds to the spleen and stomach is fine, floating, and bowstring.

How a Chinese doctor analyzes Denise's symptoms

In Chinese medicine, anger is the emotion of the liver. In Chinese, irritability is called "easy anger." So right away, the Chinese doctor suspects that liver depression qi stagnation is playing a part in Denise's PMS. This is supported by the fact that liver depression in women typically gets worse during the premenstruum due to the collection of blood in the uterus leaving the liver "high and dry" so to speak. However, Denise not only gets angry easily, she also tends to cry at little things which, at other times of the month, would not provoke such a tearful reaction. Grief and melancholy are the emotions associated with the lungs in Chinese medicine, while tears are the fluid associated with the liver, remembering that, "The liver opens into the portals of the eyes." Therefore, irritability and crying for no or little reason are typically due to some sort of pathological relationship between the liver and lungs. In addition, pathological heat tends to force body fluids to "run recklessly outside of the body." So, it is likely that it is pathological heat in the lungs which is responsible for this crying.

As we already know, if liver depression endures for a long time, it can easily transform into depressive heat. Heat, because it is yang in nature, has an innate tendency to travel upward. "The lungs are the florid canopy." This means that the lungs are the capstone of the other viscera and bowels, and so heat wafting upward from the liver below often accumulates and lodges in the lungs. This supposition is corroborated by the fact that Denise has a bitter taste in her mouth in the morning. This bitter taste is due to bile, like tears, another of the body's fluids and one which is associated with the liver. If there is depressive heat in the liver, this heat may force bile to flow recklessly upward to the mouth and thus the bitter taste.

We also know that Denise experiences premenstrual breast distention and soreness. Distention is categorized as qi stagnation and accumulation, and we have said that the qi of the chest and breasts has a special relationship with the liver. If liver qi becomes depressed and stagnant and then counterflows horizontally, it may accumulate in the breasts and chest. The fact that this liver qi has transformed in depressive heat is further corroborated by the fact that Denise's nipples get sore and inflamed premenstrually. "The liver channel homes to the nipples." Therefore, a feeling of heat in the nipples suggests depressive liver heat. Likewise, so does the premenstrual acne. The pimples are red. Red indicates heat in Chinese medicine. Pimples are a skin lesion and "The lungs govern the skin and (body) hair." Thus red skin lesions often suggest heat in the lungs. The fact that there is heat in the lungs is corroborated by the easy crying discussed above. Further, the placement of the pimples under the corners of the mouth suggest that this heat is also affecting the stomach, since this area of the face is traversed by the stomach channel. Increased appetite is another potential symptom of stomach heat, and this is corroborated by the slightly yellowish tongue fur which also indicates heat has affected the stomach. This is because the tongue fur is taken as an indication of the stomach qi and yellow as opposed to white fur indicates heat.

In addition, other signs and symptoms which add up to liver depression qi stagnation according to the logic of Chinese medicine include the premenstrual lower abdomen distention and cramping and the menstrual cramps on day one which are relieved by massage, warmth, and exercise. In Chinese medicine, it is a given that:

If there is pain, there is no free flow.
If there is free flow, there is no pain.

Since there is premenstrual and menstrual cramping, we know that the flow of qi and blood is not free and easy. Massage, warmth, and exercise all help to mobilize the qi and blood and promote free flow. Thus Denise's dysmenorrhea or painful menstruation also corroborates a Chinese pattern discrimination of liver depression qi stagnation. Likewise, Denise's periods always coming late at irregular intervals suggests that depressed qi is not allowing the blood to flow freely from the body. And finally, a bowstring pulse is "the pulse of the liver" and is the definitive pulse image denoting liver depression and constraint.

Now let's look at Denise's fatigue. W already know that the spleen is the root of qi and blood production, and fatigue is always a symptom of qi vacuity or weakness. The fact that the spleen qi in particular is weak and insufficient is corroborated first by the fact that Denise gets bloated after heavy meals. It is the spleen's job to "disperse and transform" the digestate, and, if it is weak, it cannot do this. Thus there is indigestion. Secondly, Denise's tongue is swollen and has the indentations of her teeth along its edges. The spleen is responsible for moving and transforming body fluids. If the spleen qi is weak, these body fluids accumulate and transform into dampness, thus producing a swollen, edematous tongue. Third, Denise's cravings for sweets and carbohydrates (which are metabolized into sugar) is an indication of spleen vacuity. Sweet is the flavor which "gathers" in the spleen and sweet is a "supplementing" flavor, engendering both more qi and more fluids. A little sweet flavor supplements the spleen qi, but too much actually damages the spleen further and leads to the formation of internal dampness. And finally, the floating, fine pulse in the middle position on the right wrists corresponding to the spleen also is an indication of spleen vacuity and dampness.[17]

The fact that Denise is constipated premenstrually and then has loose stools on day one of her period shows that liver depression qi stagnation is affecting her spleen function. In Chinese medical parlance, we say that the liver is assailing the spleen. Premenstrually, liver depression fails to "course and discharge" and so the stools are not discharged and precipitated. On day one, because blood is begun to be lost, the spleen becomes even weaker than it was premenstrually. This results in loose stools since spleen vacuity is one of the leading causes of diarrhea. The fact that the liver is assailing or invading the spleen is corroborated by the bowstring quality of the right middle position as well as its being floating and fine.

Therefore, based on the above signs and symptoms, the Chinese doctor knows that Denise's PMS is a combination of several factors: 1) liver depression transforming into heat, 2) depressive heat counterflowing upward and accumulating in the stomach and lungs, and 3) spleen vacuity with possibly some dampness.

How a Chinese doctor treats Denise's PMS

Once a Chinese doctor knows the patient's pattern discrimination, the next step is to formulate the treatment principles necessary to rebalance the imbalance implied by this pattern discrimination. If the Chinese doctor listed liver depression as number one in their pattern discrimination, then the first treatment principles

---

[17] Chinese doctors feel the pulse at the arteries at the styloid processes on both wrists. Each wrist is divided into three sections and each section is divided into at least two depths. Therefore, there is a total of 12 pulse positions if one counts both wrists. Each of these 12 positions corresponds to one of the five viscera or six bowels, with the kidneys having both a kidney yang and kidney yin position. By feeling a particular type of pulse in a given position, the Chinese doctor knows something about the viscus or bowel corresponding to that position.

are to course the liver and rectify the qi. These are the treatment principles for correcting liver depression qi stagnation. To course the liver means to promote the liver's coursing and discharge or spreading of the qi freely and easily throughout the body. Rectifying the qi means to make the qi move and, more than that, make it move in the right directions. If the second element in the pattern discrimination is depressive heat in the stomach and lungs, then the Chinese doctor knows that the second set of principles are to clear heat and resolve depression from those organs. And if the third element in the pattern discrimination is spleen vacuity with possible dampness, then the necessary treatment principles for rebalancing that are to fortify (*i.e.*, strengthen) the spleen and supplement the qi and possibly to eliminate dampness.

Once the Chinese doctor has stated the treatment principles, then they know that anything which works to accomplish these principles will be good for the patient. Using these principles, the Chinese doctor can now select various acupuncture points which achieve these effects. They can prescribe Chinese herbal medicinals which embody these principles. They can make recommendations about what to eat and not eat based on these principles. They can make recommendations on lifestyle changes. And, in short, they can advise the patient on any and every aspect of their life, judging whether something either aids the accomplishment of these principles or works against it.

In Chinese medicine, the internal administration of Chinese (herbal) medicinals is the main modality.[18] So let's look at how a Chinese doctor crafts a prescription for Denise. Because the liver is depressed and the spleen is weak, the Chinese doctor knows there is a disharmony between the liver and spleen. There is yet

---

[18] I've put the word herbal in parentheses since Chinese medicine is not entirely herbal. Herbs are medicinals made from parts of plants, their roots, bark, stems, leaves, flowers, etc. Chinese medicinals are mostly herbal in nature. However, a percentage of Chinese medicinals also come from the animal and mineral realms. Thus not all Chinese medicinals are, strictly speaking, herbs.

another disharmony between the spleen which is weak and the stomach which is hot. Thus the Chinese doctor knows to pick their starting formula from the "harmonizing" category of Chinese medicinal formulas.[19] Further, they need to find a harmonizing formula which courses the liver and rectifies the qi, clears heat in the stomach and lungs, and fortifies the spleen and supplements the qi.

Of the various formulas found in the harmonization chapter of the Chinese doctor's book of formulas and prescriptions, there is only one famous one which does just these things. It is called *Xiao Chai Hu Tang* (Minor Bupleurum Decoction). Let's look at its ingredients. This formula is composed of:

Radix Bupleuri *(Chai Hu)*
Radix Panacis Ginseng *(Ren Shen)*
Rhizoma Pinelliae Teranatae (*Ban Xia*)
Radix Scutellariae Baicalensis (*Huang Qin*)
mix-fried Radix Glycyrrhizae (*Gan Cao*)
Fructus Zizyphi Jujubae (*Da Zao*)
uncooked Rhizoma Zingiberis (*Sheng Jiang*)

Radix Bupleuri or Bupleurum courses the liver and rectifies the qi.[20] It is the single most used Chinese medicinal for remedying liver depression qi stagnation. Radix Panacis Ginseng or simply Ginseng is the most fmous spleen-fortifying qi supplement in

---

[19] In Chinese medicine, depending on the textbook, there are anywhere from 22-28 different categories of formulas.

[20] Because most Chinese medicinals have no commonly recognized English names, I identify these medicinals at least the first time they are introduced by first their Latin pharmacological identification followed by their Chinese name in parentheses. If the "herb" in question has a well-known common English name, the next time I refer to that ingredient, I first use the Latin followed by the common name. In subsequent instances, I then just use the common English name.

Chinese medicine.[21] However, Ginseng also quiets the spirit. Rhizoma Pinelliae Ternatae or Pinellia helps Bupleurum regulate the qi and downbear upward counterflow. At the same time, it helps Ginseng fortify the spleen. If there is any dampness, Pinellia would also transform dampness or phlegm. Radix Scutellariae Baicalensis or Scutellaria clears heat specifically from the liver, stomach, and lungs, the three organs which have accumulated depressive heat in this case. Mix-fried Radix Glycyrrhizae or Licorice helps Ginseng and Pinellia fortify the spleen and supplement the qi. In particular, Licorice supplements the spleen and heart qi. In addition, Licorice moderates any harsh actions of any of the medicinals in this formula and helps the other medicinals to act in a concerted and harmonious way. Fructus Zizyphi Jujubae or Red Dates also fortify the spleen and supplement the qi, thus aiding the other spleen supplements in this formula. Red Dates also nourish the heart blood, and, like Ginseng, help to calm the heart spirit. Uncooked Rhizoma Zingiberis or Ginger promotes the flow of qi. It also harmonizes the stomach and helps eliminate dampness as well as helps Licorice harmonize and moderate all the other ingredients.

Hence one can see that the ingredients in this formula very precisely and specifically embody and carry out the treatment principles we have said were necessary for rebalancing Denise's condition. In actual fact, this formula is the most often prescribed Chinese medicinal formula in the world. It is used to treat a very wide range of diseases *as long as the patient presents with a pattern of liver depression and spleen vacuity with heat in either*

---

[21] In this formula, it is specifically white, Chinese Ginseng which is used, not red, Korean Ginseng. Red Ginseng is warm and supplements kidney yang as well as spleen qi. Since we have not said Denise's kidney yang is weak and since we know she is already overheated, we do not want to supplement kidney yang nor add unnecessary heat. Some practitioners use the cheaper Radix Codonopsitis Pilosulae (*Dang Shen*). However, this medicinal does not quiet the heart spirit the way Ginseng does. Since Denise's spirit is vexed and not calm, using Radix Codonopsitis Pilosulae or Codonopsis is a false economy.

the liver, stomach, or lungs. This formula is not a "PMS formula" per se. It is used to treat everything from chronic bronchitis, nausea, and diarrhea to chronic tonsillitis, chronic hepatitis, and a whole host of gynecological complaints. Its choice has less to do with the disease diagnosis and everything to do with the Chinese pattern discrimination. Thus *Xiao Chai Hu Tang* does not so much treat this disease or that; it treats people with a particular set of patterns who happen to also have certain diagnosed diseases.

To make this formula even more effective, the Chinese doctor will also rarely prescribe this formula in its textbook form above. Rather, we will modify it by taking out one or more ingredients and adding others as necessary in order to tailor it to the individual patient's exact configuration of signs and symptoms. Since Denise's case is one of PMS due primarily to aggravation of liver depression premenstrually in turn due to blood collecting in the uterus leaving the liver "high and dry", I would first add Radix Angelicae Sinensis (*Dang Gui*) and Radix Albus Paeoniae Lactiflorae (*Bai Shao*). These two medicinals both nourish the blood and soften and harmonize the liver. Because they also quicken the blood, they will also help Denise's period pain. If the signs and symptoms of spleen vacuity and dampness were more pronounced, then I might add two more medicinals for fortifying the spleen and eliminating dampness: Rhizoma Atractylodis Macrocephalae (*Bai Zhu*) and Sclerotium Poriae Cocos (*Fu Ling*). If breast distention is more pronounced, I might add a couple more ingredients for rectifying or regulating the qi in the chest and breasts, such as Rhizoma Cyperi Rotundi (*Xiang Fu*) and Radix Linderae Strychnofoliae (*Wu Yao*). These should also help eliminate the period pain. If depressive heat was more ponounced, then I might add one or more medicinals for clearing heat, such as Fructus Gardeniae Jasminoidis (*Shan Zhi Zi*), Rhizoma Coptidis Chinensis (*Huang Lian*), or Herba Taraxaci Mongolici Cum Radice (*Pu Gong Ying*). This last ingredient would be a good choice because Herba Taraxaci Mongolici Cum Radice or Dandelion not only clears heat, it courses the liver qi and promotes the flow of qi specifically in the breasts. Whenever possible, we try to use the least number of ingredients which do the most of what is required. In fact, there is no limit to the modifications I might make to this formula in order to make it match perfectly Denise's exact signs and symptoms, constitution, and tolerances.

Usually, a formula such as this when used to treat PMS would be begun as soon as the PMS manifested each month and continued through the first day of the onset of the menses. The ingredients in this formula may be dispensed in bulk and then brewed as a "tea" by the patient or may be taken as a dried, powdered extract. Many standard formulas also come as ready-made pills. However, these cannot be modified. If their ingredients match the individual patient's requirements, then they are fine. If the formula needs modifications, then teas or powders whose individual ingredients can be added and subtracted are necessary.

In exactly the same way, the Chinese doctor could create an individualized acupuncture treatment plan and would certainly create an accompanying dietary and lifestyle plan. However, we will discuss each of these in their own chapter. In a woman Denise's age with her Chinese pattern discrimination, either Chinese herbal medicine alone, acupuncture alone, or a combination of the two supported by the proper diet and lifestyle will usually eliminate or at the very least drastically diminish her PMS within three months, meaning three menstrual cycles, of treatment.

Chinese Herbal Medicine & PMS

As we have seen from Denise's case above, there is no Chinese "PMS herb" or even "PMS formula." Chinese medicinals are individually prescribed based on a person's pattern discrimination, not on a disease diagnosis like PMS. Women often come to me and say, "My friend told me that Ginseng (or Dang Gui) is good for PMS. But I tried it and it didn't work." A variation of this kind of disease-oriented statement is the often heard, "Ginseng is for men and Dang Gui is for women."

If a woman has PMS and none of her symptoms are due to spleen qi vacuity, then Ginseng is not going to help that particular woman. In fact, if her pattern is liver depression transforming into heat or ascendant hyperactivity of liver yang, the woman may very well find herself having more headaches, more irritability, more red, painful eyes, and more dizziness if she takes enough Ginseng long enough. Since this woman's qi is depressed, adding more qi to what is already not flowing freely only adds to this depression which, under pressure, transforms into heat and vents itself upward to harass the head. On the other hand, if a woman with PMS does display signs and symptoms of spleen qi vacuity, then the right amount of Ginseng is "just what the doctor ordered."

Likewise, if a woman with PMS also manifests the signs and symptoms of blood vacuity or blood stasis, then taking Dang Gui will probably help relieve some of her symptoms. Dang Gui nourishes and quickens the blood. By nourishing the blood, it softens and harmonizes the liver. This does not address liver depression completely and directly, but it does help. By quickening the blood, Dang Gui does help treat pain due to blood stasis, including and especially blood stasis period pain. However, if a woman does not have much blood vacuity or blood stasis, then Dang Gui will also not have much of an effect on her PMS.

In addition, because most women's PMS is a combination of different Chinese patterns and disease mechanisms, professional Chinese medicine never treats women with PMS with herbal "singles." In herbalism, singles mean the prescription of a single herb all by itself. Chinese herbal medicine is based on rebalancing patterns, and patterns in real-life patients almost always have more than a single element. Therefore, Chinese doctors almost always prescribe herbs in multi-ingredient formulas. Such formulas may have anywhere from six to eighteen or more ingredients. When a Chinese doctor reads a prescription by another Chinese doctor, they can tell you not only what the patient's pattern discrimination is but also their probable signs and symptoms. In other words, the Chinese doctor does not just combine several medicinals which are all reputed to be "good for PMS." Rather, they carefully craft a formula whose ingredients are meant to rebalance every aspect of the patient's body–mind.

Getting your own individualized prescription

Since, in China, it takes not less than four years of full-time college education to learn how to do a professional Chinese pattern discrimination and then write an herbal formula based on that pattern discrimination, most laypeople cannot realistically write their own Chinese herbal prescriptions. It should also be remembered that Chinese herbs are not effective and safe because they are either Chinese or herbal. In fact, approximately 20% of the common Chinese materia medica did not originate in Chinese, and not all Chinese herbs are completely safe. They are only safe when prescribed according to a correct pattern discrimination, in the right dose, and for the right amount of time. After all, if an herb is strong enough to heal an imbalance, it is also strong enough to create an imbalance if overdosed or misprescribed. Therefore, I strongly recommend women who wish to experience the many benefits of Chinese herbal medicine to see a qualified professional practitioner who can do a professional pattern discrimination and write you an individualized prescription. Towards the end of this book, I will give the reader suggestions on how to find a qualified professional Chinese medical practitioner near you.

Experimenting with Chinese patent medicines

In reality, qualified professional practitioners of Chinese medicine are not yet found in every North American community. In addition, some women may want to try to heal their PMS as much on their own as possible. More and more health food stores are stocking a variety of ready-made Chinese formulas in pill and powder form. These ready-made, over the counter Chinese medicines are often referred to as Chinese patent medicines. Although my best recommendation is for women to seek Chinese herbal treatment from professional practitioners, below are some suggestions of how one might experiment with Chinese patent medicines to treat PMS.

In chapter 4, I have given the signs and symptoms of four of the key or basic patterns associated with most women's PMS. These are:

1. Liver depression qi stagnation
2. Spleen-kidney yang vacuity
3. Heart-spleen dual vacuity
4. Kidney vacuity, liver effulgence

If a woman can identify her main pattern from this chapter, then there are some Chinese patent remedies that she might consider trying.

Xiao Yao Wan (also spelled *Hsiao Yao Wan*)

Xiao Yao Wan is one of the most common Chinese herbal formulas prescribed to women suffering from PMS. Its Chinese name has been translated as Free & Easy Pills, Rambling Pills, Relaxed Wanderer Pills, and several other versions of this same idea of promoting a freer and smoother, more relaxed flow. As a patent medicine, this formula comes as pills, and there are both Chinese-made and American-made versions of this formula available over the counter in the North American marketplace.[22]

The ingredients in this formula are:

Radix Bupleuri (*Chai Hu*)
Radix Angelicae Sinensis (*Dang Gui*)
Radix Albus Paeoniae Lactiflorae (*Bai Shao*)
Rhizoma Atractylodis Macrocephalae (*Bai Zhu*)
Sclerotium Poriae Cocos (*Fu Ling*)
mix-fried Radx Glycyrrhizae (*Gan Cao*)
Herba Menthae Haplocalycis (*Bo He*)
uncooked Rhizoma Zingiberis (*Sheng Jiang*)

This formula treats the pattern of liver depression qi stagnation complicated by blood vacuity and spleen weakness with possible dampness as well. Bupleurum courses the liver and rectifies the qi. It is aided in this by Herba Menthae Haplocalycis or Peppermint. Dang Gui and Radix Albus Paeoniae Lactilforae or White Peony nourish the blood and soften and harmonize the liver. Rhizoma Atractylodis Macrocephalae or Atractylodes and Sclerotium Poriae Cocos or Poriae fortify the spleen and eliminate dampness. Mix-fried Licorice aid these two in fortifying the spleen and supplementing the liver, while uncooked Ginger aids in both promoting and regulating the qi flow and eliminating dampness.

---

[22] When marketed as a dried, powdered extract, this formula is sold under the name of Bupleurum & Tang-kuei Formula.

When PMS presents with the signs and symptoms of liver depression and spleen vacuity, one can try taking this formula as soon as any PMS symptoms appear and continue taking this formula through the first day of menstruation. However, after taking these pills at the dose recommended on the packaging, if one notices any side effects, then stop immediately and seek a professional consultation. Such side effects from this formula might include nervousness, irritability, a dry mouth and increased thirst, and red, dry eyes. Such side effects show that this formula, at least with modification, is not right for you. Although it may be doing you some good, it is also causing some harm. Remember, Chinese medicine is meant to cure without side effects, and as long as the prescription matches one's pattern there will not be any.

Dan Zhi Xiao Yao Wan

Dan Zhi Xiao Yao Wan or Moutan & Gardenia Rambling Pills is a modification of the above formula which also comes as a patent medicine in the form of pills.[23] It is meant to treat the pattern of liver depression transforming into heat with spleen vacuity and possible blood vacuity and/or dampness. The ingredients in this formula are the same as above except that two other herbs are added:

Cortex Radicis Moutan (*Dan Pi*)
Fructus Gardeniae Jasminoidis (*Shan Zhi Zi*)

These two ingedients clear heat and resolve depression. In addition, Cortex Radicis Moutan or Moutan quickens the blood and dispels stasis and is good at clearing heat specifically from the blood. Some Chinese doctors say to take out uncooked Ginger and Mint, while others leave these two ingredients in.

---

[23] When marketed as a dried, powdered extract, this formula is called Bupleurum & Peony Formula.

Basically, the signs and symptoms of the pattern for which this formula is designed are the same as those for *Xiao Yao San* above plus signs and symptoms of depressive heat. These might include a reddish tongue with slightly yellow fur, a bowstring and rapid pulse, a bitter taste in the mouth, and increased irritability.

Shu Gan Wan (also spelled *Shu Kan Wan*)

Shu Gan Wan means Soothe the Liver Pills.[24] This Chinese patent medicine is made up almost entirely of liver-coursing and qi-rectifying medicinals. Unlike *Xiao Yao Wan* above, it does not nourish the blood or supplement the spleen. Its ingredients are:

Fructus Meliae Toosendan (*Chuan Lian Zi*)
Rhizoma Curcumae Longae (*Jiang Huang*)
Lignum Aquilariae Agallochae (*Chen Xiang*)
Rhizoma Corydalis Yanhusuo (*Yan Hu Suo*)
Radix Auklandiae Lappae (*Mu Xiang*)
Semen Alpiniae Katsumadai (*Dou Kou*)
Radix Albus Paeoniae Lactiflorae (*Bai Shao*)
Sclerotium Poriae Cocos (*Fu Ling*)
Fructus Citri Aurantii (*Zhi Ke*)
Pericarpium Citri Reticulatae (*Chen Pi*)
Fructus Amomi (*Sha Ren*)
Cortex Magnoliae Officinalis (*Hou Po*)

This formula can be taken by itself when a woman's PMS really only consists of breast and abdominal distention and cramping. However, one can take these pills along with *Xiao Yao Wan* if there is liver depression and spleen and/or blood vacuity with more pronounced breast and/or abdominal distention and menstrual cramps. However, if taking these pills causes feelings of dryness or heat internally or if they make one even more vexed

---

[24] This formula does not come as a standard dried, powdered formula. However, various companies making such powdered formulas can make it as a special order.

and irritable, either their dosage should be reduced or they should be stopped.

Xiang Sha Liu Jun Wan

The name of these pills translates as Auklandia & Amomum Six Gentlemen Pills.[25] Sometimes they are referred to as Aplotaxis-Amomum Pills. This formula treats the pattern of pronounced spleen vacuity with elements of dampness and a little qi stagnation. Since the overwhelming majority of women's PMS includes liver depression qi stagnation, these pills can be taken along with *Xiao Yao Wan* in those cases where spleen vacuity is more severe. These pills are especially good for treating poor appetite, nausea, abdominal bloating after meals, and loose stools due to spleen vacuity and dampness. Their ingredients include:

Radix Codonopsitis Pilosulae (*Dang Shen*)
Rhizoma Atractylodis Macrocephalae (*Bai Zhu*)
Sclerotium Poriae Cocos (*Fu Ling*)
Rhizoma Pinelliae Ternatae (*Ban Xia*)
mix-fried Radix Glycyrrhizae (*Gan Cao*)
Pericarpium Citri Reticulatae (*Chen Pi*)
Radix Auklandiae Lappae (*Mu Xiang*)
Fructus Amomi (*Sha Ren*)

One should not take these pills, however, if there is burning around the anus with bowel movements or there is diarrhea with dark colored, foul-smelling, explosive stools.

---

[25] When sold as a dried, powdered extract, this formula is called Saussurea & Cardamon Combination.

Bu Zhong Yi Qi Wan

Bu Zhong Yi Qi Wan means Supplement the Center & Boost the Qi Pills.[26] This formula treats the pattern of central qi vacuity or central qi fall. The central qi is another name for the spleen and stomach qi. This formula is especially good for treating spleen vacuity weakness manifesting not so much as digestive complaints and diarrhea but as more pronounced fatigue and orthostatic hypotension. Orthostatic hypotension means dizziness on standing up. The ingredients in this formula are:

Radix Astaragli Membranacei (*Huang Qi*)
Radix Codonopsitis Pilosulae (*Dang Shen*)
Rhizoma Atractylodis Macrocephalae (*Bai Zhu*)
mix-fried Radix Glycyrrhizae (*Gan Cao*)
Radix Angelicae Sinensis (*Dang Gui*)
Radix Bupleuri (*Chai Hu*)
Rhizoma Cimicifugae (*Sheng Ma*)
Pericarpium Citri Reticulatae (*Chen Pi*)
Fructus Zizyphi Jujubae (*Da Zao*)
uncooked Rhizoma Zingiberis (*Sheng Jiang*)

This is acutally a very sophisticated formula and it has a very wide range or application. Because it includes Bupleurum and Dang Gui, it courses the liver and rectifies the qi as well as nourishes the blood and softens the liver. It can be added to *Xiao Yao Wan* when spleen vacuity causing fatigue is more pronounced. Since spleen vacuity typically does become more pronounced after the age of 35, these pills are often the guiding prescription or are combined with other formulas.

---

[26] When sold as a dried, powdered extract, this formula is called Ginseng & Astragalus Combination.

Ba Zhen Wan

Ba Zhen Wan literally means Eight Pearls Pills.[27] However, these are also often marketed under the name Women's Precious Pills. They are called "eight pearls" because they include four ingredients which supplement the qi and four ingredients which nourish the blood. These pills can be combined with *Xiao Yao Wan* when there is liver depression complicated by more serious spleen qi and liver blood vacuity. Their ingredients are:

Radix Codonopsitis Pilosulae (*Dang Shen*)
Rhizoma Atractylodis Macrocephalae (*Bai Zhu*)
Sclerotium Poriae Cocos (*Fu Ling*)
mix-fried Radix Glycyrrhizae (*Gan Cao*)
Radix Angelicae Sinensis (*Dang Gui*)
Radix Albus Paeoniae Lactiflorae (*Bai Shao*)
cooked Radix Rehmanniae (*Shu Di*)
Radix Ligustici Wallichii (*Chuan Xiong*)

Shi Quan Da Bu Wan

The name of these pills translates as Ten (Ingredients) Completely & Greatly Supplementing Pills.[28] Their ingredients are the same as *Ba Zhen Wan* above plus:

Cortex Cinnamomi Cassiae (*Rou Gui*)
Radix Astragali Membranacei (*Huang Qi*)

Basically they are the same formula. Some Chinese doctors feel that these extra two ingredients help the body generate new qi and blood more rapidly. Therefore, it can be added to *Xiao Yao*

---

[27] When sold as a dried, powdered extract, this formula is called Tang-kuei & Ginseng Eight Combination.

[28] When sold as a dried, powdered extract, this formula is called Ginseng & Tang-kuei Ten Combination.

Wan for the same reasons as *Ba Zhen Wan*. However, because Cortex Cinnamomi Cassiae or Cinnamon Bark is hot, it should not be used if there is depressive heat. In other words, one would not usually combine these pills with *Dan Zhi Xiao Yao Wan*.

Tabellae *Suan Zao Ren Tang*

This is a tableted version of the formula, *Suan Zao Ren Tang* (Zizyphus Seed Decoction).[29] It treats insomnia and mental unrest due to liver blood vacuity. It can, therefore, be combined with *Xiao Yao Wan* when liver blood vacuity is more severe and manifests primarily as insomnia. Its ingredients are:

Semen Zizyphi Spinosae (*Suan Zao Ren*)
Sclerotium Poriae Cocos (*Fu Ling*)
Radix Ligustici Wallichii (*Chuan Xiong*)
Rhizoma Anemarrhenae Aspheloidis (*Zhi Mu*)
mix-fried Radix Glycyrrhizae (*Gan Cao*)

Gui Pi Wan (also spelled *Kuei Pi Wan*)

Gui means to return or restore, *pi* means the spleen, and *wan* means pills. Therefore, the name of these pills means Restore the Spleen Pills.[30] However, these pills not only supplement the spleen qi but also nourish heart blood and calm the heart spirit. They are the textbook guiding formula for the pattern of heart-spleen dual vacuity. In this case, there are symptoms of spleen qi vacuity, such as fatigue, poor appetite, and cold hands and feet plus symptoms of heart blood vacuity, such as a pale tongue, heart palpitations, and insomnia. This formula is also the standard one for treating heavy or abnormal bleeding due to the spleen not

---

[29] When sold as a dried, powdered extract, this formula is called Zizyphus Combination.

[30] When sold as a dried, powdered extract, this formula is called Ginseng & Longan Combination.

containing and restraining the blood within its vessels. Therefore, this patent medicine can be combined with *Xiao Yao San* when there is liver depression qi stagnation complicated by heart blood and spleen qi vacuity. Its ingredients are:

Radix Astragali Membranacei (*Huang Qi*)
Radix Codonopsitis Pilosulae (*Dang Shen*)
Rhizoma Atractylodis Macrocephalae (*Bai Zhu*)
Sclerotium Parardicis Poriae Cocos (*Fu Shen*)
mix-fried Radix Glycyrrhizae (*Gan Cao*)
Radix Angelicae Sinensis (*Dang Gui*)
Semen Zizyphi Spinosae (*Suan Zao Ren*)
Arillus Euphoriae Longanae (*Long Yan Rou*)
Radix Polygalae Tenuifoliae (*Yuan Zhi*)
Radix Auklandiae Lappae (*Mu Xiang*)

Er Chen Wan

Er Chen Wan means Two Aged (Ingredients) Pills.[31] This is because two of its main ingredients are aged before using. This formula is used to transform phlegm and eliminate dampness. It can be added to *Xiao Yao Wan* if there is liver depression with spleen vacuity and more pronounced phlegm and dampness. Its ingredients include:

Rhizoma Pinelliae Ternatae (*Ban Xia*)
Sclerotium Poriae Cocos (*Fu Ling*)
mix-fried Radix Glycyrrhizae (*Gan Cao*)
Pericarpium Citri Reticulatae (*Chen Pi*)
uncooked Rhizoma Zingiberis (*Sheng Jiang*)

---

[31] When sold as a dried, powdered extract, this formula is called Citrus & Pinellia Combination.

Ge Jie Da Bu Wan

Gecko Greatly Supplementing Pills supplement the qi, blood, yin, and yang. It is usually used to treat low back and lower limb pain associated with kidney vacuity in turn due to aging. Because most women develop not only spleen vacuity but also kidney yin and yang vacuity as they move towards menopause in their late 40s, this formula can be combined with *Xiao Yao Wan* when there is liver depression, spleen and kidney yang vacuity, and blood and yin vacuity as well. The ingredients in this Chinese patent medicine include:

Gecko (*Ge Jie*)
Radix Astragali Membranacei (*Huang Qi*)
Radix Codonopsitis Pilosulae (*Dang Shen*)
Fructus Lycii Chinensis (*Gou Qi Zi*)
Radix Angelicae Sinensis (*Dang Gui*)
cooked Radix Rehmanniae (*Shu Di*)
Fructus Ligustri Lucidi (*Nu Zhen Zi*)
Rhizoma Polygonati (*Huang Jing*)
Rhizoma Atractylodis Macrocephalae (*Bai Zhu*)
Sclerotium Poriae Cocos (*Fu Ling*)
Radix Dioscoreae Oppositae (*Shan Yao*)
Radix Glycyrrhizae (*Gan Cao*)
Cortex Eucommiae Ulmoidis (*Du Zhong*)
Radix Dipsaci (*Xu Duan*)
Rhizoma Cibotii Barmetsis (*Gou Ji*)
Radix Morindae Officinalis (*Ba Ji Tian*)
Rhizoma Drynariae (*Gu Sui Bu*)
Fructus Chaenomelis Lagenariae (*Mu Gua*)

Jiang Ya Wan (also spelled *Chaing Ya Wan*)

Jiang Ya means to decrease pressure as in high blood pressure. *Wan* as we've seen before means pills. These pills are usually used to treat high blood pressure due to kidney vacuity and liver effulgence. The reader should remember that actually Chinese medicine treats patterns of imbalance, not diseases such as high blood pressure. Also remember the saying, "Different diseases, same treatment." Therefore, these pills can be used to treat PMS complaints such as headaches, including migraines, dizziness, red, painful eyes, and irritability due to an upward flaring of liver fire or wind in turn due to loss of control by kidney yin below. Since this formula already includes medicinals for treating the liver, it would not be combined with *Xiao Yao Wan* above but used by itself. Its ingredients are:

Semen Leonuri Heterophyli (*Chong Wei Zi*)
Rhizoma Coptidis Chinensis (*Huang Lian*)
Cornu Antelopis Saiga-tatarici (*Ling Yang Jiao*)
Spica Prunellae Vulgaris (*Xia Ku Cao*)
Ramulus Uncariae Cum Uncis (*Gou Teng*)
Radix Gastrodiae Elatae (*Tian Ma*)
Succinum (*Hu Po*)
Raix Angelicae Sinensis (*Dang Gui*)
Radix Ligustici Wallichii (*Chuan Xiong*)
uncooked Radix Rehmanniae (*Sheng Di*)
Gelatinum Corii Asini (*E Jiao*)
Cortex Radicis Moutan (*Dan Pi*)
Radix Achyranthis Bidentatae (*Niu Xi*)
Lignum Aquilariae Agallochae (*Chen Xiang*)
Radix Et Rhizoma Rhei (*Da Huang*)

Because this formula contains Radix Et Rhizoma Rhei or Rhubarb which is a strong purgative, it should not be taken if one has diarrhea or loose stools. If this formula causes diarrhea, its use should be discontinued.

The above Chinese patent medicines only give a suggestion of how one or several over the counter Chinese ready-made preparations may be used to treat PMS. As a professional practitioner of Chinese medicine, I prefer to see women receive a professional diagnosis and an individually tailored prescription. However, as long as one is careful to try to match up their pattern with the right formula and not to exceed the recommended dosage, one can try treating their PMS with one or more of these remedies. If it works, great! These patent medicines are usually quite cheap. If this approach doesn't work after three cycles or if there are *any side effects*, one should stop and see a professional practitioner.

In general, you can tell if any medication and treatment are good for you by checking the following six guideposts.

1. Digestion
2. Elimination
3. Energy level
4. Mood
5. Appetite
6. Sleep

If a medication, be it modern Western or traditional Chinese, gets rid of your symptoms and all six of these basic areas of human health improve or are fine to begin with, then that medicine or treatment is probably OK. However, even if a treatment or medication takes away your major complaint, if it causes deterioration in one of these six basic parameters, then that treatment or medication is probably not OK and is certainly not OK for long–term use. When medicines and treatments, even so-called natural, herbal medications, are prescribed based on a person's pattern of disharmony, then there is healing without side effects. According to Chinese medicine, this is the only kind of true healing.

Acupuncture & Moxibustion

When the average Westerner thinks of Chinese medicine, they probably first think of acupuncture. Certainly acupuncture is the best known of the various methods of treatment which go to make up Chinese medicine. However, in China, acupuncture is actually a secondary treatment modality, most Chinese immediately thinking of "herbal" medicine when thinking of Chinese medicine.

Be that as it may, most professional practitioners of Chinese medicine in North America are licensed or otherwise registered and permitted to practice medicine as acupuncturists. Therefore, most such practitioners treat every patient with at least some acupuncture no matter if they also prescribe a Chinese herbal formula as well. While this "doubling up" of these two therapies is not always necessary to successfully treat most women's PMS, PMS in general does respond very well to correctly prescribed and administered acupuncture.

What is acupuncture?

Acupuncture primarily means the insertion of extremely thin, sterilized, stainless steel needles into specific points on the body where Chinese doctors have known for centuries there are special concentrations of qi and blood. Therefore, these points are like switches or circuit breakers for regulating and balancing the flow of qi and blood over the channel and network system we described above. As we have seen, PMS complaints are called menstrual movement diseases in Chinese medicine. This means that they are diseases due to the erroneous flow of the qi and blood prior to the menses. As we have also seen, there really is no PMS if there is not also liver depression, and liver depression means that the qi is stagnant. Because the qi is depressed and stagnant, it is not flowing when and where it should. Instead it counterflows or vents itself to areas of the body where it shouldn't be, attacking other organs and body tissues and making them dysfunctional.

Therefore, PMS typically includes many signs and symptoms associated with lack of, or errroneous, counterflow qi flow. Since acupuncture's forte is the regulation and rectification of the flow of qi (and, thus secondarily, the blood), it is an especially good treatment mode for correcting menstrual movement diseases. In that case, insertion of acupuncture needles at various points in the body moves stagnant qi in the liver and leads the qi to flow in its proper directions and amounts.

As a generic term, acupuncture also includes several other methods of stimulating acupuncture points, thus regulating the flow of qi in the body. The main other modality is moxibustion. This means the warming of acupuncture points mainly by burning dried, aged Oriental mugwort on, near, or over acupuncture points. The purpose of this warming treatment are to 1) even more strongly stimulate the flow of qi and blood, 2) add warmth to areas of the body which are too cold, and 3) add yang qi to the body to supplement a yang qi deficiency. Other acupuncture modalities are to apply suction cups over points, to massage the points, to prick the points to allow a drop or two of blood to exit, to apply Chinese medicinals to the points, to apply magnets to the points, and to stimulate the points by either electricity or laser.

What is a typical acupuncture treatment for PMS like?

In China, acupuncture treatments are given every other day, three times a week beginning from the first day of the onset of any PMS signs or symptoms. This means that treatment would begin on day 21 if the woman's symptoms began on day 21, while it might begin on day 17 in another woman whose symptoms began on day 17. Once the symptoms appear, then treatment is given every other day through the first day of menstruation. This regime is then repeated again the next month. However, if the treatment has been correct and if the woman has been following her practitioner's advice about diet, exercise, lifestyle, and relaxation, then her symptoms should start later and later each month. This means that she should need less and less treatments each month.

When the woman comes for her appointment, the practitioner will ask her what her main symptoms are, will typically look at her tongue and its fur, and will feel the pulses at the radial arteries on both wrists. Then, they will ask the woman to lie down on a treatment table. Based on their Chinese pattern discrimination, the practitioner will select anywhere from one to eight or nine points to be needled.

The needles used today are ethylene oxide gas sterilized disposable needles. This means that they are used one time and then thrown away, just like a hypodermic syringe in a doctor's office. However, unlike relatively fat hypodermic needles, acupuncture needles are hardly thicker than a strand of hair. The skin over the point is disinfected with alcohol and the needle is quickly and deftly inserted somewhere typically between one quarter and a half inch. In some few cases, a needle may be inserted deeper than that, but most needles are only inserted relatively shallowly.

After the needle has broken the skin, the acupuncturist will usually manipulate the needle in various ways until he or she feels that the qi has "arrived." This refers to a subtle but very real feeling of resistance around the needle. When the qi arrives, the patient will usually feel a mild, dull soreness around the needle, a slight electrical feeling, a heavy feeling, or a numb or tingly feeling. All these mean that the needle has tapped the qi and that treatment will be effective. Once the qi has been tapped, then the practitioner may further adjust the qi flow by manipulating the needle in certain ways, may attach the needle to an electro-acupuncture machine in order to stimulate the point with very mild and gentle electricity, or they may simply leave the needle in place. Usually the needles are left in place from 10-20 minutes. After this, the needles are withdrawn and thrown away. *Thus there is absolutely no chance for infection from another patient.*

How are the points selected?

The points one's acupuncturist chooses to needle each treatment are selected on the basis of Chinese medical theory and the known clinical effects of certain points. Since there are different schools or styles of acupuncture, point selection tends to vary from practitioner to practitioner. However, let me present a fairly typical case from the point of view of the dominant style of acupuncture in the People's Republic of China.

Let's say the woman's main complaints are premenstrual breast distention and pain but no lumps or cystic tissue, irritability, fatigue, and loose stools. Her tongue is fat and pale with thin, slightly slimy, white fur, and her pulse is fine and bowstring. Her Chinese pattern discrimination is premenstrual breast distention and pain, easy anger, and fatigue due to liver depression and spleen vacuity. This is a very commonly encountered Chinese pattern of disharmony in women with PMS up to approximately 35 years of age.

The treatment principles necessary for remedying this case are to course the liver and rectify the qi, fortify the spleen and supplement the qi. In addition, because breast distention and pain are major complaints, the practitioner will add the treatment principles of loosen the chest and free the flow in the breasts. In order to accomplish these aims, the practitioner might select the following points:

Tai Chong (Liver 3)
San Yin Jiao (Spleen 6)
Zu San Li (Stomach 36)
Ru Gen (Stomach 18)
Shan Zhong (Conception Vessel 17)
Pi Shu (Bladder 20)
Wei Shu (Bladder 21)

In this case, *Tai Chong* courses the liver and resolves depression, moves and rectifies the qi. Since liver depression qi stagnation is the main disease mechanism causing this woman's PMS, this is the main or ruling point in this treatment. Since this woman's easy anger or irritability stems from liver depression, this point also eliminates the source of this woman's vexation.

San Yin Jiao is chosen to further course the liver at the same time as it fortifies the spleen. It does both these things because both the liver and spleen channels cross at this point. In addition, this point is known to be empirically effective for most genitourinary and reproductive diseases. In Chinese medicine, it is said to possess a menstrual-regulating effect.

Zu San Li is the most powerful point on the stomach channel. Because the stomach is yang and the spleen is yin and because the stomach and spleen share a mutually "exterior/interior" relationship, stimulating *Zu San Li* can bolster the spleen with yang qi from the stomach which usually has plenty. In addition, the stomach channel traverses the chest and, therefore, needling this point can regulate the qi in the chest and breasts in general.

Ru Gen is also a point on the stomach channel. However, it is located just under the breasts and is a main "local" point for freeing and regulating the flow of qi through the breasts. Likewise, *Shan Zhong*, which is located at the level of the nipples on the chest bone between the breasts, is also a local point for freeing the flow of qi in the chest and breasts. This point is a special point for regulating the flow of qi in the entire body, but especially in the chest. It also helps calm the spirit and provide emotional relief.

Pi Shu and *Wei Shu* are both points on the back associated with the spleen and stomach respectively. They directly connect with this viscus and bowel and can supplement weakness and deficiencies in these two organs. In particular, this woman's fatigue and loose stools both stem from spleen vacuity, and these two points are known to empirically address both of these complaints.

Thus this combination of seven points addresses this woman's Chinese pattern discrimination and her major complaints of breast distention and soreness, irritability, and fatigue and loose stools. It remedies both the underlying disease mechanism and addresses certain key symptoms in a very direct and immediate way. Hence it provides symptomatic relief *at the same time as* it corrects the underlying mechanisms of these symptoms.

Does acupuncture hurt?

In Chinese, it is said that acupuncture is *bu tong*, painless. However, most patients will feel some mild soreness, heaviness, electrical tingling, or distention. When done well and sensitively, it should not be sharp, biting, burning, or really painful.

How quickly will I feel the result?

One of the best things about the acupuncture treatment of PMS is that its effects are immediate. Since many of the symptoms of PMS have to do with stuck qi, as soon as the qi is made to flow, the symptoms disappear. Therefore, for many PMS complaints, such as breast distention and pain, headache, low back pain, lower abdominal cramps, joint or muscle pain, or epigastric pain, *one will feel relief during the treatment itself.*

In addition, because irritability and nervous tension are also mostly due to liver depression qi stagnation, most women will feel an immediate relief of irritability and tension while still on the table. Typically, one will feel a pronounced tranquility and relaxation within five to ten minutes of the insertion of the needles.

Who should get acupuncture?

As mentioned above, because most professional practitioners in the West are legally entitled to practice under various acupuncture laws, most acupuncturists will routinely do acupuncture on every patient. Since acupuncture's effects on PMS are usually so immediate, this is usually a good thing for PMS sufferers. However, acupuncture is particularly effective for breast distention and pain, and even if one is prescribed Chinese herbal medicinals for premenstrual breast complaints, one should consider a course of acupuncture in addition. Because acupuncture treats pain so effectively and immediately, one should consider receiving acupuncture especially for any PMS complaints associated with pain. And because acupuncture treats mental-emotional tension so well and so immediately, women with PMT should also get at least one course of acupuncture therapy.

When a woman's PMS symptoms mostly have to do with qi vacuity, blood vacuity, or yin vacuity, then acupuncture is not as effective as internally administered Chinese herbal medicinals. Although moxibustion can add yang qi to the body (and I will teach a home remedy for this in a separate section on moxibustion below), acupuncture needles cannot add qi, blood, or yin to a body in short supply of these. The best acupuncture can do in these cases is to stimulate the various viscera and bowels which engender and transform the qi, blood, and yin. Chinese herbs, on the other hand, can directly introduce qi, blood, and yin into the body, thus supplementing vacuities and insufficiencies of these. In PMS cases, where qi, blood, and yin vacuities are pronounced, one should either use acupuncture with Chinese medicinals or rely on

Chinese medicinals alone. When there is pronounced yang vacuity, one can use moxibustion alone or with Chinese medicinals, but one should not use needles alone.

Ear acupuncture

Acupuncturists believe there is a map of the entire body in the ear and that by stimulating the corresponding points in the ear, one can remedy those areas and functions of the body. Therefore, many acupuncturists will not only needle points on the body at large but also select one or more points on the ear. In terms of PMS, ear acupuncture is especially good for two things. First, needling the point *Shen Men* (Spirit Gate) can have a profound effect on relaxing tension and irritability and improving sleep. Secondly, needling the Mouth and/or Stomach points, one can decrease and control overeating and various cravings.

The nice thing about ear acupuncture points is that one can use tiny "press needles" which are shaped like miniature thumbtacks. These are pressed into the points, covered with adhesive tape, and left in place for five to seven days. This method can provide continuous treatment between regularly scheduled office visits. Thus ear acupuncture is a nice way of extending the duration of an acupuncture treatment. In addition, these ear points can also be stimulated with small metal pellets, radish seeds, or tiny magnets, thus getting the benefits of stimulating these points without having to insert actual needles.

The Three Free Therapies

Although one can experiment cautiously with Chinese herbal medicinals, one cannot really do acupuncture on oneself. Therefore, Chinese herbal medicine and acupuncture and its related modalities mostly require the aid of a professional practitioner. However, there are three free therapies which are crucial to preventing and treating PMS. These are diet, exercise, and deep relaxation.

Remember that the root cause of PMS is liver depression qi stagnation. This is then typically complicated by spleen vacuity weakness. Liver depression is primarily due to stress and emotional factors, while spleen vacuity is primarily due to faulty diet. Of these three free therapies, therefore, diet is designed to cure the spleen, and exercise and relaxation are meant to cure the liver. When all three are coordinated, then they eliminate the causes and disease mechanisms of most women's PMS. Since Western women's diets are, by Chinese medical standards, typically poor and since Western society tends to be both excessively sedentary and excessively stressful, lack of proper management of these three basic realms of human life is the reason why so many Western women suffer from PMS. In other words, although PMS has been around for millenia, its incidence is probably higher now in the West because of relatively recent changes in our diet and lifestyle.

Diet

In Chinese medicine, the function of the spleen and stomach are likened to a pot on a stove or still. The stomach receives the foods and liquids which then "rotten and ripen" like a mash in a fermentation vat. The spleen then cooks this mash and drives off (*i.e.*, transforms and upbears) the pure part. This pure part collects in the lungs to become the qi and in the heart to become the blood. In addition, Chinese medicine characterizes this transformation as a process of yang qi transforming yin substance. All the principles of Chinese dietary therapy, including what women with PMS should and should not eat, are derived from these basic "facts."

We have seen that a healthy spleen is vitally important for keeping the liver in check and the qi freely flowing. We have also seen that the spleen is the root of qi and blood transformation and engenderment. Therefore, it is vitally important for women with PMS to avoid foods which damage the spleen and to eat foods which promote a healthy spleen and qi and blood production.

Foods which damage the spleen

In terms of foods which damage the spleen, Chinese medicine begins with uncooked, chilled foods. If the process of digestion is likened to cooking, then cooking is nothing other than predigestion outside of the body. In Chinese medicine, it is a given that the overwhelming majority of all food should be cooked, *i.e.*, predigested. Although cooking may destroy some vital nutrients (in Chinese, qi), cooking does render the remaining nutrients much more easily assimilable. Therefore, even though some nutrients have been lost, the net absorption of nutrients is greater with cooked foods than raw. Further, eating raw foods makes the spleen work harder and thus wears the spleen out more quickly. If one's spleen is very robust, eating uncooked, raw foods may not be so damaging, but we have already seen that many women's spleens are already weak because of their monthly menses overtaxing the spleen *vis à vis* blood production.

More importantly, chilled foods directly damage the spleen. Chilled, frozen foods and drinks neutralize the spleen's yang qi. The process of digestion is the process of warming all foods and drinks to 100° Fahrenheit within the stomach so that it may undergo transformation. If the spleen expends too much yang qi just warming the food up, then it will become damaged and weak. Therefore, all foods and liquids should be eaten and drunk at room temperature at the least and better at body temperature. The more signs and symptoms of spleen vacuity a woman presents, such as fatigue, chronically loose stools, undigested food in the stools, cold hands and feet, dizziness on standing up, and aversion to cold, the more closely she should avoid uncooked, chilled foods and drinks.

In addition, sugars and sweets directly damage the spleen. This is because sweet is the flavor which inherently "enters" the spleen. It is also an inherently dampening flavor according to Chinese medicine. This means that the body engenders or secretes fluids which gather and collect, transforming into dampness, in response to foods with an excessively sweet flavor. In Chinese medicine, it is said that the spleen is averse to dampness. Dampness is yin and controls or checks yang qi. The spleen's function is based on the transformative and transporting functions of yang qi. Therefore, anything which is excessively dampening can damage the spleen. The sweeter a food is, the more dampening and, therefore, more damaging it is to the spleen.

Another group of foods which are dampening and, therefore, damaging to the spleen is what Chinese doctors call "sodden wheat foods." This means flour products such as bread and noodles. Wheat (as opposed to rice) is damp by nature. When wheat is steamed, yeasted, and/or refined, it becomes even more dampening. In addition, all oils and fats are damp by nature and, hence, may damage the spleen. The more oily or greasy a food is, the worse it is for the spleen. Because milk contains a lot of fat, dairy products are another spleen-damaging, dampness-engendering food. This includes milk, butter, and cheese.

If we put this all together, then ice cream is just about the worst thing a woman with a weak, damp spleen could eat. Ice cream is chilled, it is intensely sweet, and it is filled with fat. Therefore, it is a triple whamy when it comes to damaging the spleen. Likewise, pasta smothered in tomato sauce and cheese is a recipe for disaster. Pasta made from wheat flour is dampening, tomatoes are dampening, and cheese is dampening. In addition, what many women don't know is that a glass of fruit juice contains as much sugar as a candy bar, and, therefore, is also very damaging to the spleen and damp-engendering.

Below is a list of specific Western foods which are either uncooked, chilled, too sweet, or too dampening and thus damaging to the spleen. Women with PMS should minimize or avoid these proportional to how weak and damp their spleen is.

Ice cream	Juicy, sweet fruits, such as
Sugar	oranges, peaches, strawberries,
Candy, especially chocolate	and tomatoes
Milk	Fatty meats
Butter	Fried foods
Cheese	Refined flour products
Margarine	Yeasted bread
Yogurt	Nuts
Raw salads	Alcohol (which is essentially
Fruit juices	sugar)

If the spleen is weak and wet, one should also not eat too much at any one time. A weak spleen can be overwhelmed by a large meal, especially if any of the food is hard-to-digest. This then results in food stagnation which only impedes the free flow of qi all the more and further damages the spleen.

A clear, bland diet

In Chinese medicine, the best diet for the spleen and, therefore, by extension for most humans, is what is called a "clear, bland diet." This is a diet high in complex carbohydrates such as unrefined grains, especially rice, and beans. It is a diet which is high in *lightly cooked* vegetables. It is a diet which is low in fatty meats, oily, greasy, fried foods, and very sweet foods. However, it is not a completely vegetarian diet. Most women, in my experience should eat one to two ounces of various types of meat two to four times per week. This animal flesh may be the highly popular but overtouted chicken and fish, but should also include some lean beef, pork, and lamb. Some fresh or cooked fruits may be eaten, but fruit juices should be avoided. In addition, women should make an effort to include tofu and tempeh, two soy foods now commonly available in North American grocery food stores.

If the spleen is weak, then one should eat several smaller meals than one or two large meals. In addition, because rice is 1) neutral in temperature, 2) it fortifies the spleen and supplements the qi, and 3) it eliminates dampness, rice should be the main or staple grain in the diet.

A few problem foods

There are a few "problem" foods which desrve special mention. The first of these is coffee. Many women crave coffee for two reasons. First, coffee moves stuck qi. Therefore, if a woman suffers from liver depression qi stagnation, temporarily coffee will make her feel like her qi is flowing. Secondly, coffee transforms essence into qi and makes that qi temporarily available to the body. Therefore, women who suffer from spleen and/or kidney vacuity fatigue will get a temporary lift from coffee. They will feel like they have energy. However, once this energy is used up, they are left with a negative deficit. The coffee has transformed some of the essence stored in the kidneys into qi. This qi has been used, and now there is less stored essence. Since the blood and essence share a common source, coffee drinking may ultimately worsen PMS associated with blood or kidney vacuities. Since the kidneys are linked with the *chong* vessel and chronic breast diseases are associated with disharmonies of this vessel, coffee drinking can cause or aggravate breast diseases associated with the *chong* vessel.

Another problem food is chocolate. Chocolate is a combination of oil, sugar, and cocoa. We have seen that both oil and sugar are dampening and damaging to the spleen. Temporarily, the sugar will boost the spleen qi, but ultimately it will result in "sugar blues" or a hypoglycemic let-down. Cocoa stirs the life gate fire. The life gate fire is another name for kidney yang or kidney fire, and kidney fire is the source of sexual energy and desire. It is said that chocolate is the food of love, and from the Chinese medical point of view, that is true. Since chocolate stimulates kidney fire at the same time as it temporarily boosts the spleen, it does give one rush of yang qi. In addition, this rush of yang qi does move depression and stagnation, at least short-term. So it makes sense that some women with liver depression, spleen vacuity, and kidney yang debility might crave chocolate premenstrually.

Alcohol is both damp and hot according to Chinese medical theory. It strongly moves the qi and blood. Therefore, persons with liver depression qi stagnation will feel temporarily better from drinking alcohol. However, the sugar in alcohol damages the spleen and engenders dampness which "gums up the works," while the heat (yang) in alcohol can waste the blood (yin) and aggravate or inflame depressive liver heat.

Spicy, peppery, "hot" foods also move the qi, thereby giving some temporary relief to liver depression qi stagnation. However, like alcohol, the heat in spicy hot foods wastes the blood and can inflame yang.

In Chinese medicine, the sour flavor is inherently astringing and constricting. Therefore, women with PMS should be careful not to use vinegar and other intensely sour foods premenstrually. Such sour flavored foods will only aggravate the qi stagnation by astringing and restricting the qi and blood all the more. This is also why sweet and sour foods, such as orange juice and tomatoes are particularly bad for women with liver depression/spleen vacuity PMS. The sour flavor astringes and constricts the qi, while the sweet flavor damages the spleen and engenders dampness.

In my experience, diet sodas seem to contain something that damages the Chinese idea of the kidneys. They may not damage the spleen the same way that sugared sodas do, but that does not mean they are healthy and safe. I say that diet sodas damage the kidneys since a number of my patients over the years have reported that, when they drink numerous diet sodas, they experience terminal dribbling, urinary incontinence, and low back and knee soreness and weakness. When they stop drinking diet sodas, these symptoms disappear. Taken as a group, in Chinese medicine, these are kidney vacuity symptoms. Since women with PMS in their late 30s and throughout their 40s tend to suffer from concomitant kidney vacuity (along with liver depression and spleen vacuity), I typically recommend such women to steer clear of diet sodas so as not to weaken their kidneys any further or faster.

Candidiasis & PMS

If one looks at the foods which I have recommended to minimize or avoid above and what I have recommended women with PMS to eat, one will see that it comes very close or is identical to an anti-candida diet. Polysystemic chronic candidiasis (PSCC) refers to a chronic overgrowth of yeasts and fungi in the body which then goes on to affect many different systems in the body. The pathological changes associated with PSCC are due to a combination of food allergies, immune system dysregulation, and autoimmune reactions. In women, these pathological changes may affect the ovaries, adrenals, pituitary gland, and thyroid gland. In Western women, a tendency towards PSCC is due to faulty diet as outlined above, overuse of antibiotics, and overuse of hormone-based medicine from oral birth control pills to corticosteroids. From a Chinese medical point of view, this then results in deep-seated spleen vacuity with damp encumberance possibly complicated by liver depression, phlegm fluids, damp heat, and/or blood stasis. If the spleen vacuity lasts long enough or due to aging, spleen vacuity may also involve kidney yang vacuity.

If a woman with PMS has a history of multiple fungal and yeast infections, a history of recurrent or enduring antibiotic use (such as for recurrent bladder infections or pelvic inflammatory disease), has a history of hormones used as medicine, or suffers from allergies, PSCC should be suspected as a component of that woman's PMS. In that case, the woman should pay particular attention to her diet. The good news is that professionally prescribed Chinese herbal medicine can help remedy PSCC faster than just diet alone. The bad news is that, without proper diet, no amount of Chinese herbs will completely and permanently remedy this condition.

Vitamins

The Western popular press has published numerous articles on the benefits of taking various Western nutritional supplements for PMS. The main one of these is vitamin B_6. Strictly speaking, such vitamin therapy is not a part of traditional Chinese medicine. However, even in China, patients routinely take Western vitamins and nutritional supplements along with Chinese herbs. Therefore, women should feel free to take such Western vitamins and Western nutritional supplements along with Chinese herbal medicine. However, some Western nutritionists recommend women to take various fatty acids for PMS, such as flax seed oil. Although this may benefit some women's PMS, it will cause problems with others.

In particular, women with weak spleens should be careful about taking fatty acids for their PMS. As we have seen, oils are dampening and can easily damage the spleen. In my experience as a clinician, if one experiences nausea or vomiting, indigestion or loose stools after taking such fatty acids, then these side effects are because these oils have caused further dampening of the spleen. In this case, the right person has not taken the right supplement. This is exactly the strong point of Chinese medicine and one of the major themes of this book. Chinese medicine allows the patient and their practitioner to determine if any treatment or food will be good or bad for them on the basis of their individualized pattern discrimination. As all women know, one size does not fit all!

Some last words on diet

In conclusion, many women with PMS ask me what they should eat in order to cure their PMS. However, when it comes to diet, sad to say, the issue is not so much what to eat as what not to eat. There are, in my experience, no magic foods which cure PMS. Diet most definitely plays a major role in the cause and perpetuation of most women's PMS, but the issue is mainly what to avoid or minimize, not what to eat. Most of us know that coffee, chocolate, sugars and sweets, oils and fats, and alcohol are not good for us. Most of us know that we should be eating more complex carbohydrates and freshly cooked vegetables and less fatty meats. However, it's one thing to know these things and another to follow what we know.

To be perfectly honest, a clear bland diet *à la* Chinese medicine is not the most exciting diet in the world. It is the traditional diet of most lower and lower middle class peoples around the world living in temperate climates. It is the traditional diet of most of my readers' great grandparents. The point I am making here is that our modern Western diet which is high in oils and fats, high in sugars and sweets, high in animal proteins, and proportionally high in uncooked, chilled foods and drinks is a relatively recent aberration, and you can't fool Mother Nature.

When one switches to the clear, bland diet of Chinese medicine, at first one may suffer from cravings for more "flavorful" food. These cravings are, in many cases, actually associated with food "allergies." In other words, we may crave what is actually not good for us similar to a drunk's craving alcohol. After a few days, these cravings tend to disappear and we may be amazed that we don't miss some of our convenience or "comfort" foods as much as we thought we would. If one has been addicted to a food like sugar for many years, it does not take much to "fall off the wagon" and be addicted again. Therefore, perserverance is the key to long-term success. As the Chinese say, a million is made up of nothing but lots of ones, and a bucket is quickly filled by steady drips and drops.

Exercise

Exercise is the second of what I call the three free therapies. According to Chinese medicine, regular and adequate exercise has two basic benefits. First, exercise promotes the movement of the qi and quickening of the blood. Since all PMS involves at least some component of liver depression qi stagnation, it is obvious that exercise is an important therapy for coursing the liver and rectifying the qi. Secondly, exercise benefits the spleen. The spleen's movement and transportation of the digestate is dependent upon the qi mechanism. The qi mechanism describes the function of the qi in upbearing the pure and downbearing the turbid parts of digestion. For the qi mechanism to function properly, the qi must be flowing normally and freely. Since exercise moves and rectifies the qi, it also helps regulate and rectify the qi mechanism. This then results in the spleen's movement and transportation of foods and liquids and its subsequent engendering and transforming of the qi and blood. Because spleen and qi and blood vacuity typically complicate most women's PMS and because a healthy spleen checks and controls a depressed liver, exercise treats the other most commonly encountered disease mechanism in the majority of Western women's PMS. Therefore, it is easy to see that regular, adequate exercise is a vitally important component of any woman's regime for either preventing or treating PMS.

What kind of exercise is best for PMS?

In my experience, I find aerobic exercise to be the most beneficial for most women with PMS. By aerobic exercise, I mean any physical activity which raises one's heartbeat 80% above their normal resting rate and keeps it there for at least 20 minutes. To calculate your normal resting heart rate, place your fingers over the pulsing artery on the front side of your neck. Count the beats for 15 seconds and then multiply by four. This gives you your beats per minute or BPM. Now multiply your BPM by 0.8. Take the resulting number and add it to your resting BPM. This gives you your aerobic threshold of BPM. Next engage in any physical activity you like. After you have been exercising for five minutes, take your pulse for 15 seconds once again at the artery on the front side of your throat. Again multiply the resulting count by four and this tells you your current BPM. If this number is less than your aerobic threshold BPM, then you know you need to exercise harder or faster. Once you get your heart rate up to your aerobic threshold, then you need to keep exercising at the same level of intensity for at least 20 minutes. In order to insure that one is keeping their heartbeat high enough for long enough, one should recount their pulse every five minutes or so.

Depending on one's age and physical condition, different women will have to exercise harder to reach their aerobic threshold than others. For some women, simply walking briskly will raise their heartbeat 80% above their resting rate. For other women, they will need to do calisthenics, running, swimming, racketball, or some other, more stenuous exercise. It really does not matter what the exercise is as long as it raises your heartbeat 80% above your resting rate and keeps it there for 20 minutes. However, there are two other criteria that should be met. One, the exercise should be something that is not too boring. If it is too boring, then you may have a hard time keeping up your schedule. Since most people do find aerobic exercises such as running, stationary bicycles, and stair-steppers boring, it is good to listen to music or watch TV in order to distract your mind from the tedium. Secondly, the type of exercise should not cause any damage to any parts of the body. For instance, running on pavement may cause knee problems for some people. Therefore, you should pick a type of exercise you enjoy but also one which will not cause any problems.

When doing aerobic exercise, it is best to exercise either every day or every other day. If one does do their aerobics at least once every 72 hours, then its cumulative effects will not be as great. Therefore, I recommend my PMS patients to do some sort of aerobic exercises every day or every other day, three to four times per week *at least*. The good news is that there is no real need to exercise more than 30 minutes at any one time. Forty-five minutes per session is not going to be all that much better than 25 minutes per session. And 25 minutes four times per week is much better than one hour once a week.

Recent research has also demonstrated that weight-lifting can help relieve depression in women of all ages.[32] Therefore, I have begun recommending lifting weights on the days when one is not doing aerobics. In that case, one can do aerobics three to four days a week and lift weights the other three days. In general, one should not lift weights every day unless one varies the muscle groups they are working each day. In the study on weight-lifting and depression cited above, the women lifted weights which were 45-87% as heavy as the maximum they could lift at one time. Those women who lifted weights closer to the top end of this range saw the greatest benefits. These women lifted weights three days

---

[32] "Depression and Weight Training", *Harvard Women's Health Watch*, Vol. IV, #6, February 1997, reporting on research published in the *Journal of Gerontology*, January 1997

per week for 10 weeks, gradually increasing the amount of weight they lifted at each session.

Because weight-lifting requires some initial training and education in order to do it safely and properly, I recommend taking a few classes either at a local YMCA or recreation center or from a private trainer. When aerobics are alternated with weight-lifting, one has a really comprehensive training regime designed to benefit both one's cardiovascular system and one's muscles, tendons, ligaments, and bones. In addition, regular weight-bearing exercise is also important for preventing osteoporosis.

Deep relaxation

As we have seen above, PMS is associated with liver depression qi stagnation. Typically, the worse the PMS is, the worse the woman's liver depression. In Chinese medicine, liver depression comes from not fulfilling all one's desires. But as we have also seen above, no adult can fulfill all their desires. This is why a certain amount of liver depression is endemic among adults. When our desires are frustrated, our qi becomes depressed. This then creates emotional depression and easy anger or irritability. In Chinese medicine, anger is nothing other than the venting of pent up qi in the liver. When qi becomes depressed in the liver, it accumulates like hot air in a ballon. Eventually, that hot, depressed, angry qi has to go somewhere. So when there is a little more frustration or stress, then this angry qi in the liver vents itself as irritability, anger, shouting, or nasty words.

Essentially, this type of anger and irritability are due to a maladaptive coping response that is typically learned at a young age. When we feel frustrated or stressed, stymied by or angry about something, most of us tense our muscles and especially the muscles in our upper back and shoulders, neck, and jaws. At the same time, many of us will hold our breath. In Chinese medicine, the sinews are governed by the liver. This tensing of the muscles, *i.e.*, the sinews, constricts the flow of qi in the channels and network vessels. Since it is the liver which is responsible for the coursing and discharging of this qi, such tensing of the sinews leads to liver depression qi stagnation. Because the lungs govern the downward spreading and movement of the qi, holding our breath due to stress or frustration only worsen this tendency of the qi not to move and, therefore, to become depressed in the Chinese medical idea of the liver.

Therefore, deep relaxation is the third of the three free therapies. For deep relaxation to be therapeutic medically, it needs to be more than just mental equilibrium. It needs to be somatic or bodily relaxation as well as mental repose. Most of us no longer recognize that every thought we think and feeling we feel is actually a felt physical sensation somewhere in our body. The words we use to describe emotions are all abstract nouns, such as anger, depression, sadness, and melancholy. However, in Chinese medicine, *every emotion is associated with a change in the direction or flow of qi*. For instance, anger makes the qi move upward, while fear makes it move downward. Therefore, anger "makes our gorge rise" or "blow our top", while fear may cause a "sinking feeling" or make us "pee in our pants." These colloquial expressions are all based on the age-old wisdom that all thoughts and emotions are not just mental but also bodily events. This is why it is not just enough to clear one's mind. Clearing one's mind is good, but for really marked therapeutic results, it is even better if one clears one's mind at the same time as relaxing every muscle in the body as well as the breath.

Guided deep relaxation tapes

The single most efficient and effective way I have found for myself and my patients to practice such mental and physical deep relaxation is to do a daily, guided, progressive, deep relaxation audiotape. What I mean by guided is that a narrator on the tape leads one through the process of deep relaxation. Such tapes are progressive since they lead one through the body in a progressive manner, first relaxing one body part and then moving on to another. For instance, the narrator may say something to the effect that, as you exhale, you should feel your forehead get heavy and relaxed, softening and expanding, becoming warm and heavy. As you exhale again, now feel your cheeks get heavy and relaxed, softening and expanding, becoming warm and heavy. Breathe in and breathe out, letting your breath go without hinderance or hesitation. Breathing out, now feel your jaw muscles become heavy and relaxed, expanding and softening, becoming warm and heavy, etc., etc. throughout the entire body until one comes to the bottoms of one's feet.

There are innumerable such tapes on the market. These are usually sold in health food stores, New Age music and supply stores, or in bookstores with a good selection of New Age books. Over the years of suggesting this method of deep relaxation to my patients, I have found that each patient will have her own preferences in terms of the type of voice, male or female, the choice of words and imagery, whether there is background music or not, and the actual pace of the progression through the body. Therefore, I suggest listening to and even purchasing more than one such tape. One should find a tape which they like and can listen to without internal criticism or comment, going along like a cloud in the sky as the narrator's voice blows away all your mental and bodily stress and tension. If one has more than one tape, one can also switch every now and again from tape to tape so as not to become bored with the process or desensitized to the instructions.

Key things to look for in a good relaxation tape

In order to get the full therapeutic effect of such deep relaxation tapes, there are several key things to check for. First, be sure that the tape is a guided tape and not a subliminal relaxation tape. Subliminal tapes usually have music and any instructions to relax are given so quietly that they are not consciously heard. Although such tapes can help you feel relaxed when you do them, ultimately they do not teach you how to relax as a skill which can be consciously practiced and refined. Secondly, make sure the tape starts from the top of the body and works downward. Remember, anger makes the qi go upward in the body, and people with irritability and easy anger due to liver depression qi stagnation already have too much qi rising upward in their bodies. Such depressed qi typically needs not only to be moved but also downborne. Third, make sure the tape instructs you to relax your physical body. If you do not relax all your muscles or sinews, the qi cannot flow freely and the liver cannot be coursed. Depression is not resolved, and there will not be the same medically therapeutic effect. And lastly, be sure the tape instructs you to let your breath go with each exhalation. One of the symptoms of liver depression is a stuffy feeling in the chest which we then unconsciously try to relieve by sighing. Letting each exhalation go completely helps the lungs push the qi downward. This allows the lungs to control the liver at the same time as it downbears upwardly counterflowing angry liver qi.

The importance of daily practice

When I was an intern in Shanghai in the People's Republic of China, I was once taken on a field trip to a hospital clinic where they were using deep relaxation as a therapy with patients with high blood pressure, heart disease, stroke, and migraines. The doctors at this clinic showed us various graphs plotting their research data on how such daily, progressive deep relaxation can regulate the blood pressure and body temperature and improve the appetite, digestion, elimination, sleep, energy, and mood. One of the things they said has stuck with me for 15 years: "Small results in 100 days, big results in 1,000." This means that if one does such daily, progressive deep relaxation *every single day for 100 days*, one will definitely experience certain results. What are these "small" results? These small results are improvements in all the parameters listed above: blood pressure, body temperature, appetite, digestion, elimination, sleep, energy, and mood. If these are "small" results, then what are the "big" results experienced in

1,000 days of practice? The "big" results are a change in how one reacts to stress—in other words, a change in one's very personality or character.

What these doctors in Shanghai stressed and what I have also experienced both personally and with my patients is that it is vitally important to do such daily, guided, progressive deep relaxation every single day, day in and day out for a solid three months at least and for a continuous three years at best. If one does such progressive, somatic deep relaxation every day, one will see every parameter or measurement of health and well-being improve. If one does this kind of deep relaxation only sporadically, missing a day here and there, it will feel good when you do it, but it will not have the marked, cumulative therapeutic effects it can. Therefore, perserverance is the real key to getting the benefits of deep relaxation.

The real test

Doing such a daily deep relaxation regime is like hitting tennis balls against a wall or hitting a bucket of balls at a driving range. It is only practice; it is not the real game itself. Doing a daily deep relaxation regime is not only in order to relieve one's immediate stress and strain. It is to learn a new skill, a new way to react to stress. The ultimate goal is to learn how to breathe out and immediately relax all one's muscles in the body in reaction to stress, rather than the common but unhealthy maladaption to stress of holding one's breath and tensing one's muscles. By doing such deep relaxation day after day, you will learn how to relax any and every muscle in your body quickly and efficiently. Then, as soon as you recognize that you are feeling frustrated, stressed out, or uptight, you can immediately remedy those feelings at the same time as coursing your liver and rectifying your qi. This is the real test, the game of life. "Small results in 100 days, big results in 1,000."

Finding the time

If you're like me and most of my patients, you are probably asking yourself right now, "All this is well and good, but when am I supposed to find the time to eat well-balanced cooked meals, exercise at least every other day, and do a deep relaxation every day? I'm already stretched to the breaking point." I know. That's the problem.

As a clinician, I often wish I could wave a magic wand over my patients' heads and make them all healthy and well. I cannot. After close to two decades of working with thousands of patients, I know of no easy way to health. There is good living and there is easy living. Or perhaps I am stating this all wrong. What most people take as the easy way these days is to continue pushing their limits continually to the max. The so-called path of least resistance is actually the path of lots and lots of resistance. Unless you take time for yourself and find the time to eat well, exercise, and relax, no treatment is going to eliminate your PMS completely. There is simply no pill you can pop or food your can eat that will get rid of the root causes of PMS: poor diet, too little exercise, and too much stress. Even Chinese herbal medicine and acupuncture can only get their full effect if the diet and lifestyle is first adjusted. Sun Si-maio, the most famous Chinese doctor of the Tang dynasty (618-907 CE), who himself refused government office and lived to be 101, said: "First adjust the diet and lifestyle and only secondarily give herbs and acupuncture." Likewise, it is said today in China, "Three parts treatment, seven parts nursing." This means that any cure is only 30% due to medical treatment and 70% is due to nursing, meaning proper diet and lifestyle.

In my experience, this is absolutely true. Seventy percent of all disease will improve after three months of proper diet, exercise, relaxation, and lifestyle modification. Seventy percent! Each of us has certain nondiscretionary rituals we perform each day. For instance, you may always and without exception find the time to brush your teeth. Perhaps it is always finding the time to shower.

For others, it may be always finding the time each day to eat lunch. And for 99.99% of us, we find time, no, we make the time to get dressed each day. The same applies to good eating, exercise, and deep relaxation. Where there's a will there's a way. If your PMS is bad enough, you can find the time to eat well, get proper exercise, and do a daily deep relaxation tape.

The solution to PMS is in your hands

In Boulder, CO where I live, we have a walking mall in the center of town. On summer evenings, my wife and I often walk down this mall. Having treated so many patients over the years, it is not unusual for me to meet former patients on these strolls. Frequently when we say hello, these patients begin by telling me they are sorry they haven't been in to see me in such a long time. They usually say this apologetically as if they have done something wrong. I then usually ask if they've been alright. Often they tell me: "When my such-and-such flares up, I remember what you told me about my diet, exercise, and lifestyle. I then go back to doing my exercise or deep relaxation or I change my diet, and then my symptoms go away. That's why I haven't been in. I'm sorry."

However, such patients have no need to be sorry. This kind of story is music to my ears. When I hear that these patients are now able to control their own conditions by following the dietary and lifestyle advice I gave them, I know that, as a Chinese doctor, I have done my job correctly. In Chinese medicine, the inferior doctor treats disease after it has appeared. The superior doctor prevents disease before it has arisen. If I can teach my patients how to cure their symptoms themselves by making changes in their diet and lifestyle, then I'm approaching the goal of the high class Chinese doctor—the prevention of disease through patient education.

109

The professional practice of medicine is a strange business. We doctors are always or at least should be engaged in putting ourselves out of business. Therefore, patients have no need to apologize to me when they tell me they now have control over their health and disease in their own hands.

To get these benefits, one must make the necessary changes in eating and behavior. In addition, PMS is not a condition that is cured once and forever like measles or mumps. When I say Chinese medicine can cure PMS, I do not mean that you will never experience premenstrual symptoms again. What I mean is that Chinese medicine can eliminate or greatly reduce your symptoms *as long as you keep your diet and lifestyle together*. People being people, we all "fall off the wagon" from time to time and we all "choose our own poisons." I do not expect perfection from either my patients or myself. Therefore, I am not looking for a lifetime cure. Rather, I try to give my patients an understanding of what causes their disease and what they can do to minimize or eliminate its causes and mechanisms. It is then up to the patient to decide what is bearable and what is unbearable or what is an acceptable level of health. The Chinese doctor will have done their job when *you know how to correct your health to the level you find acceptable given the price you have to pay*.

Simple Home Remedies for PMS

Although faulty diet, lack of adequate exercise, and too much stress are the ultimate causes of PMS according to Chinese medicine and, therefore, diet, exercise, and deep relaxation are the most important parts of every woman's treatment and prevention of PMS, there are a number of simple Chinese home remedies to help relieve the symptoms of PMS.

Chinese aromatherapy

In Chinese medicine, the qi is seen as a type of wind or vapor. The Chinese character for qi shows wind blowing over a rice field. In addition, smells are often referred to as a thing's qi. Therefore, there is a close relationship between smells carried through the air and the flow of qi in a person's body. Although aromatherapy has not been a major part of professionally practiced Chinese medicine for almost a thousand years, there is a simple aromatherapy treatment which one can do at home which can help alleviate premenstrual irritability, depression, nervousness, anxiety, and insomnia.

In Chinese, *Chen Xiang* means "sinking fragrance." It is the name of Lignum Aquilariae Agallochae or Eaglewood. This is a frequent ingredient in Asian incense formulas. In Chinese medicine, Aquilaria is classified as a qi-rectifying medicinal. When used as a boiled decoction or "tea", Aquilaria moves the qi and stops pain, downbears upward counterflow and regulates the middle (*i.e.*, the spleen and stomach), and promotes the kidneys' grasping of the qi sent down by the lungs. I believe that the word sinking in this herb's name refers to this medicinal's downbearing of upwardly counterflowing qi. Such upwardly counterflowing eventually must accumulate in the heart, disturbing and causing restlessness of the heart spirit. When this medicinal wood is burnt and its smoke is inhaled as a medicinal incense, its downbearing and spirit-calming function is emphasized.

One can buy Aquilaria or *Chen Xiang* from Chinese herb stores in Chinatowns, Japantowns, or Koreatowns in major urban areas. One can also buy it from Chinese medical practitioners who have their own pharmacies. It is best to use the powdered variety. However, powder may be made by putting a small piece of this aromatic wood in a coffee grinder. It is also OK to use small bits of the wood if powder is not available. Next one needs to buy a roll of incense charcoals. Place one charcoal in a nonflammable dish and light it with a match. Then sprinkle a few pinches of Aquilaria powder on the lit charcoal. As the smoke rises, breathe in deeply. This can be done on a regular basis one or more times per day during the premenstruum or on an as-needed basis by those suffering from restlessness, nervousness, anxiety, irritability, and depression. For those who experience premenstrual insomnia, one can do this "treatment" when lying in bed at night.

This Chinese aromatherapy with Lignum Aquilariae Agallochae is very cheap and effective. I know of no side effects or contraindications.

Magnet therapy

The Chinese have used magnet therapy since at least the Tang dynasty (618-907 CE). Placing magnets on the body is a safe and painless way of stimulating acupuncture points without inserting needles through the skin. Since magnets can be taped onto points and "worn" for days at a time, Chinese magnet therapy is able to provide easy, low cost, continuous treatment. Below are magnetic treatments for menstrual irregularities, including early, delayed, and erratic menstruation, excessive and scanty menstruation, lower abdominal pain occurring either before or at the onset of the period, and premenstrual breast distention and pain. Special adhesive magnets for stimulating acupuncture points, such as Accu-Band Magnets, Corimag, or Epaule Patch TDK Magnets, may be purchased from Oriental Medical Supply Co. located at 1950 Washington St., Braintree, MA 02184; Tel: (617) 331-3370 or 800-323-1839; Fax: (617) 335-5779. These range in strength from 400-9,000 gauss, the unit measuring magnetic strength. For the treatments below, one can try 400-800 gauss magnets.

Magnet therapy for menstrual irregularities

Tape small body magnets over the following points with the south pole in contact with the skin if the condition is due to liver depression qi stagnation, depressive liver heat, or blood stasis. Place the north pole against the skin if the condition is due to spleen, liver, or kidney vacuities. Leave the magnets in place for three to five days at a time. Then remove for one day so that the body does not become habituated to this stimulation and reapply for another three to five days as needed.

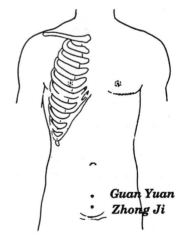

Guan Yuan (Conception Vessel 4): This point is located on the midline of the lower abdomen four finger breadths below the navel. It connects directly to both the kidneys and the uterus.

Zhong Ji (Conception Vessel 3): This point is located on the midline of the lower abdomen five finger breadths below the navel. It also connects with the uterus.

113

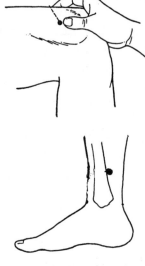

Xue Hai (Spleen 10): This point is located approximately two inches above the upper, inside edge of the kneecap when the knee is bent. This point's name means Sea of Blood and so it is used to treat all blood diseases, especially heat in the blood and static blood.

San Yin Jiao (Spleen 6): This point is located three inches above the tip of the inner ankle bone on the back edge of the tibia or lower leg bone. It is an intersection point of the spleen, liver, and kidney channels which all enter the uterus. It is used to treat all genitourinary and reproductive tract disorders. It has a very broad regulating action on menstruation.

In case of breast distention and pain, add *Gan Shu* (Bladder 18). This point is located one and a half inches lateral to the center of the spine at the same level as the lower edge of the ninth thoracic vertebra. This point connects directly with the liver and is used to treat diseases due to liver patterns of disharmony.

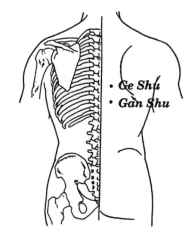

In case of early menstruation with purplish blood clots due to depressive heat and blood stasis, add *Ge Shu* (Bladder 17). This point is located one and a half inches lateral to the center of the spine at the same level as the lower edge of the seventh thoracic vertebra.

Magnet therapy for pre- & menstrual lower abdominal pain

Tape small body magnets over the following points. In case of repletion patterns of liver depression, damp heat, depressive heat, and blood stasis, the south pole should touch the skin. In case of vacuity patterns of the spleen, liver, and/or kidneys, the north pole should touch the skin. Apply three days before the expected onset of the period and leave in place until after the time the menstrual pain would ordinarily have ceased.

Guan Yuan (Conception Vessel 4): See p. 113)
Zhong Ji (Conception Vessel 3): See p.113)

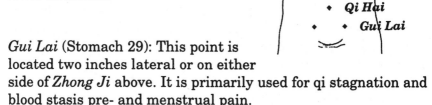

Qi Hai (Conception Vessel 6):
This point is located two finger
breadths below the navel on the
midline of the lower abdomen.
Its name means Sea of Qi and
it governs the qi of the entire
body and especially of the
lower abdomen.

Gui Lai (Stomach 29): This point is
located two inches lateral or on either
side of *Zhong Ji* above. It is primarily used for qi stagnation and blood stasis pre- and menstrual pain.

San Yin Jiao (Spleen 6): See p. 114.

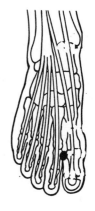

In case of qi stagnation, add *Xing Jian*
(Liver 2). This point is located just
above the web between the large and
second toes on the top of the foot. It
is the drainage point of the liver and
thus drains liver depression qi
stagnation and depressive liver heat.

115

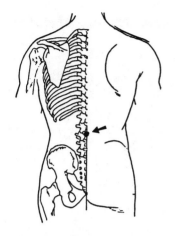

In case of vacuity cold, add *Ming Men* (Governing Vessel 4). This point is located in the center of the spine just below the lower edge of the second lumbar vertebra. *Ming Men* means life gate and refers to the life gate fire or kidney yang. Thus this point supplements the kidneys and invigorates yang. The north side of the magnet should generally touch the skin at this point.

In case of early menstruation with purplish blood clots due to blood heat and stasis, add *Ge Shu* (Bladder 17). See above.

Magnet therapy for premenstrual breast distention & pain and fibrocystic breasts

Tape small body magnets over the following points. Since most breast disease is at least locally a repletion or excess condition, tape the south sides in contact with the skin. Leave in place for three to five days. Then remove and take a rest for one day so as to prevent the body from habituating to the stimulation. Then reapply as needed.

Jian Jing (Gallbladder 21): This point is located at the high point in the top center of the trapezius or shoulder muscle. It strongly downbears upwardly counterflowing qi.

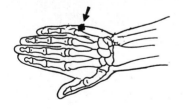

HouXi (Small Intestine 3): This point is located on the side of the hand below the little finger where the "heart line" meets the back of the hand. This point is known to have a very strong empirical effect on breast diseases due to counter-flowing qi in turn due to depression.

Ru Gen (Stomach 18): This point is located directly beneath the nipple in the fifth inter-costal space. It frees the flow of qi locally in the breasts and is used for a variety of breast diseases.

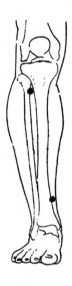

Zu San Li (Stomach 36): This point is located three inches below the lower, outside edge of the kneecap. It regulates the qi of the entire body and especially of the stomach channel which traverses the breasts.

San Yin Jiao (Spleen 6): Point three inches above inner ankle bone shown at left. See also p. 114.

If there are any cystic lumps, also tape a magnet with the south side touching the skin directly over these.

Light therapy

Light therapy, more specifically sunbathing or heliotherapy, is one of Chinese medicine's health preservation and longevity practices. Sunlight is considered the most essential yang qi in nature. Li Shi-zhen, one of the most famous Chinese doctors of the late Ming dynasty (1368-1644 CE) wrote, *"Tai yang* (literally, supreme yang but a name for the sun) is true fire." As he pointed out, "Without fire, heaven is not able to engender things, and

117

without fire, people are not able to live." Because the back of the human body is yang (as compared to the front which is more yin), exposing the back to sunlight is a good way of increasing one's yang qi.

As we have seen above, most women's yang qi begins to decline by around 35 years of age. In women over 35 years of age, most premenstrual fatigue, loose stools, lack of strength, poor memory, lack of concentration, poor coordination, decline in or lack of libido, low back and knee soreness and weakness, increased nighttime urination, and cold hands and feet are due to this decline first in the yang qi of the spleen and later in the yang qi of the spleen and kidneys. When many women say they are depressed, what they mean in Chinese medical terms is that they are extremely fatigued. In such cases, sunbathing can help supplement the yang qi of the body, thereby strengthening the spleen and/or kidneys.

Furthermore, because the yang qi is also the motivating force which pushes the qi, increasing yang qi can also help resolve depression and move stagnation. Cao Ting-dong, a famous doctor of the Qing dynasty (1644-1911 CE) wrote:

> Sitting with the back exposed directly to the sun, the back may get warmed. This is able to make the entire body harmonious and smoothly flowing. The sun is the essence of *tai yang* and its light strengthens the yang qi of the human body.

In Chinese medicine, whenever the words harmonious and smoothly flowing are used together, they refer to the flow of qi and blood. Hence sunbathing can help course the liver and rectify the qi as well as fortify the spleen and invigorate the kidneys.

It has been said that sunlight is good for every disease except skin cancer. As we now know, overexposure to the sun can cause skin cancer due to sunlight damaging the cells of the skin. Therefore, one should be careful not to get too much sun and not to get burnt. In Chinese medicine, sunbathing should be done between the hours of 8-10 AM. One should only sunbathe between 11 AM-1 PM in winter in temperate, not tropical, latitudes.

It is interesting to note that some Western researchers are coming to understand that exposure to light does play a role in many women's PMS.

Hydrotherapy

Hydrotherapy means water therapy and is a part of traditional Chinese medicine. There are numerous different water treatments for helping relieve various symptoms of PMS. First, let's begin with a warm bath. If one takes a warm bath just slightly higher than body temperature for 15-20 minutes, this can free and smooth the flow of qi and blood. In addition, it can calm the spirit and hasten sleep. Taking a warm bath a half hour before going to bed can help premenstrual insomnia. It can also relieve premenstrual tension and irritability.

However, when using a warm bath, one must be careful not to use water so hot or to stay in the bath so long that sweat breaks out on one's forehead. We lose yang qi as well as body fluids when we sweat. Because "fluids and blood share a common source", excessive sweating can cause problems for women with blood and yin vacuities. Sweating can also worsen yang qi vacuities in women whose spleen and kidneys are weak. Therefore, unless one is given a specific hot bath prescription by their Chinese medical practitioner, I suggest women with PMS not stay in warm baths until they sweat. Although they may feel pleasantly relaxed, they may later feel excessively fatigued or excessively hot and thirsty. The later is especially the case in women who are peri-menopausal. In these women, hot baths may increase hot flashes and night sweats.

If, due to depression transforming heat, yang qi is exuberant and counterflowing upward, it may cause premenstrual migraines and

119

tension headaches, hot flashes, night sweats, painful, red eyes, or even nosebleeds. In this case, one can tread in cold water up to their ankles for 15-20 minutes at a time. One may also soak their hands in cold water. Or they may put cold, wet compresses on the backs of their necks. The first two treatments seek to draw yang qi away from the head to either the lower part of the body or out to the extremities. The third treatment seeks to block and neutralize yang qi from counterflowing upward, congesting in the head and damaging the blood vessels in the head.

For women who either catch cold before each period or who are struggling with obesity, one can use cool baths slightly lower than body temperature for 10 minutes per day. Although this may seem contradictory, since cold is yin and these patients already suffer from a yang insufficiency, this brief and not too extreme exposure to cool water stimulates the body to produce more yang qi. In the case of premenstrual colds and flus, I would only do this treatment after ovulation and up to the onset of the menses. In the case of obesity due to a low metabolic rate, one can do such cool baths from the cessation of menstruation to its onset. In Chinese medicine, it is not advisable to take cold baths during the menstruation itself as this may retard the free flow of qi and blood and lead to dysmenorrhea or painful menstruation.

For painful menstruation due to qi stagnation and blood stasis, one can apply warm, wet compresses to the lower abdomen for 15-20 minutes at a time. One should not sleep with a hot water bottle or heating pad. If one uses such a hot application for too long, it begins to raise the body temperature. The body must maintain its normal temperature of 98.6° F. Therefore, if the body temperature goes up due to local application of heat, the body's response is to actually cut off the blood flow to that area of the body. This then would result in just the opposite, unwanted effect.

Likewise warm, wet compresses can be applied to the breasts for the relief of premenstrual breast distention and pain. In either case, painful menstruation or breast distention and pain, cooking several slices of fresh ginger in the water at a low boil for five to seven minutes and then using the resulting "tea" to make the hot compress can increase the compresses effect of moving the qi and quickening the blood.

Chinese self-massage

Massage, including self-massage, is a highly developed part of traditional Chinese medicine. At its most basic, rubbing promotes the flow of qi and blood in the area rubbed. Below are three Chinese self-massage regimes. The first is for headache, the second for menstrual irregularities in general, and the third for premenstrual breast distention and pain. In fact, there are Chinese self-massage regimes for diarrhea, constipation, nausea and vomiting, acne, all sorts of body pain, colds and flus, insomnia, dizziness, and painful menstruation. All of these may be used premenstrually by women with PMS. For more Chinese self-massage regimes, the reader should see Fan Ya-li's *Chinese Self-massage Therapy: The Easy Way to Health*, also published by Blue Poppy Press.

Self-massage for headache

Begin by pressing and kneading the area between the eyebrows above the bridge of the nose. This is the acupuncture point *Yin Tang* (M-HN-3) and is especially useful for calming the spirit and soothing the liver. Do this approximately 100 times.

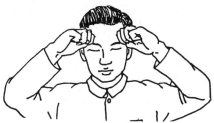

Next, rub the eyebrows with the thumbs and forefingers from the center outward. Do this 100 times.

121

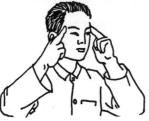

Third, rub the temples with the tips of the thumbs or middle fingers 100 times until there is a feeling of mild soreness and distention.

Fourth, rub the temples backward with the edges of the thumbs, from the orbits of the eyes to within the hairline 100 times. Only rub in one direction—from front to back.

Fifth, place the fingers of one hand on the forehead so that the middle finger is in the middle of the forehead and the other fingers are just below the hairline to either side. The palm of the hand will be resting gently on the top of the head. Now massage backward from the forehead to the center of the top of the head 20-30 times. The hands should move backward by grasping and relaxing the fingertips.

Sixth, pat the top of the head with the hollow of the palm 30-50 times. The point in the middle of the top of the head is called *Bai Hui* (Meeting of Hundreds, Governing Vessel 20). Stimulation of this point calms the spirit and downbears upwardly counter-flowing and exuberant liver yang.

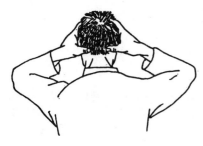

Seventh, press and knead the base of the skull in the depressions on both sides of the back of the neck. This is acupuncture point *Feng Chi* (Gallbladder 20) and is a major point for relieving headache due to upwardly counterflowing liver qi. Do this approximately 100 times.

122

And lastly, lightly pound the center of the top of one shoulder with the fist of the opposite hand. This is acupuncture point *Jian Jing* (Gallbladder 21). It also downbears upwardly counterflowing liver qi. Do this 30-50 times on each side.

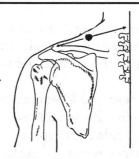

This self-massage regime is appropriate for premenstrual migraines and other types of headaches due to the upward counterflow of liver yang, depressive heat, or liver wind and/or fire.

Self-massage for menstrual irregularities

Menstrual irregularities refers to early menstruation, delayed menstruation, erratic menstruation, excessive menstruation, and scanty menstruation. It can also be used for premenstrual spotting and premenstrual lower abdominal bloating and pain.

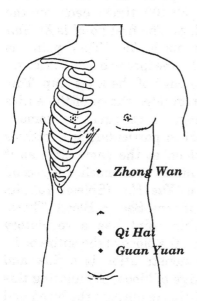

Begin by pressing and kneading each of three points 100 times. First press and knead *Zhong Wan* (Conception Vessel 12). This point is located on the midline of the abdomen, halfway between the lower tip of the sternum and the navel. Next press and knead *Qi Hai* (Conception Vessel 6). This point is on the midline of the lower abdomen, two finger breadths below the navel. Then press and knead *Quan Yuan* (Conception Vessel 4). This point is located four finger breadths below the navel on the midline of the lower abdomen. *Zhong Wan* regulates the spleen and stomach, the root of qi and blood

123

engenderment and transformation. *Qi Hai* regulates the qi in the entire body and especially in the uterus. *Guan Yuan* also connects directly to the uterus and regulates menstruation.

Next, press and knead all down the large muscles on either side of the spine. Press and knead approximately one and a half inches on either side of the spine. There are acupuncture points along the spine which connect directly with all the viscera and bowels. The production and function of the qi and blood is dependent on the proper functioning of the viscera and bowels and regular menstruation depends on the proper production and function of the qi and blood.

Third, press and knead the sacrum. Points on the sacrum connect directly with the uterus and so regulate menstruation.

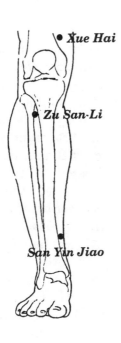

Fourth, press and knead three points 50-100 times each on the lower legs. The first point is *Zu San Li* (Stomach 36). This point is located three inches below the lower, outside edge of the knee-cap. This point regulates the qi of the entire body, regulates the qi of the stomach channel in particular, and fortifies the spleen at the same time as it harmonizes the stomach. The second point is *Xue Hai* (Spleen 10). Its name means Sea of Blood. Therefore, this point has a regulatory effect on the blood of the entire body. Since menstruation is a flow and discharge of blood, stimulating this point helps to quicken the blood and dispel stasis. It is located approxi-

124

mately two inches above the upper, inside edge of the kneecap when the knee is bent. The third point is *San Yin Jiao* (Spleen 6). This point is an intersection of the spleen, liver, and kidney channels, all three of which connect directly with the uterus. It is used for all genitourinary and reproductive tract diseases. It is located three inches above the tip of the inner anklebone on the back edge of the tibia or lower leg bone.

Fifth, rub and pat the low back or lumbar region. First rub the lumbar region back and forth from side to side until the area becomes warm to the touch. Then pat the area with the hollow of both palms 30-50 times. "The low back is the mansion of the kidneys", and this stimulates the kidneys, remembering that kidney essence is required to make blood and the kidneys connect directly to the uterus.

Finally, rub the ribs with both palms in a downward angle from the armpits to the center of the upper abdomen until this area becomes warm to the touch. Then rub from the lower edges of the ribcage to the midpoint of the lower abdomen until this area gets warm. And lastly, rub from the navel down to the pubic bone, in one direction only, five to ten times.

Self-massage for premenstrual breast distention & pain

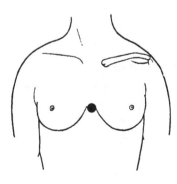

Begin by gently massaging any lumps within the breasts for 10 min-utes. Then press and knead the cen-ter of the breastbone between the nipples. This is acupuncture point *Shan Zhong* (Conception Vessel 17). It regulates all the qi in the body and especially chest and breast qi. It also calms the spirit. Do this 100-200 times.

Next, knead the underarms with the tips of the middle fingers, first one underarm and then the other. Do this 100 times on each side.

Then push the breasts with both palms simultaneously. Push lightly from every side of the breasts towards the nipples for three to five minutes.

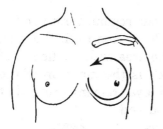

Fourth, rub the breasts lightly in circles. First rub the circles from the outside to the inside. Then reverse directions and rub from inside to outside. Do this until the breasts feel warm.

Fifth, rub the sides of the chest from the armpits downward to the center of the upper abdomen the same as in the last step of the self-massage for menstrual irregularities above. Do this until these areas feel warm.

Finally, rub the abdomen in a circle in a clockwise direction around the navel for approximately five minutes.

The key to success with Chinese self-massage therapy is perserverance. Although a single massage may provide some symptomatic relief on that very day, it is repeated self-massage day after day which can make stable and lasting changes.

Flower therapy

People have been bringing other people flowers for millenia to help them feel good. In Chinese medicine, there is actually a practice of flower therapy. Because the beauty of flowers bring most people joy and because joy is the antidote to the other four or seven negative emotions of Chinese medicine, flowers can help promote the free and easy flow of qi. It is said in Chinese medicine that, "Joy leads to relaxation (in the flow of qi)", and relaxation is exactly what the doctor ordered in cases of premenstrual liver depression qi stagnation. As Wu Shi-ji wrote in the Qing dynasty, "Enjoying flowers can divert a person from their boredom and alleviate suffering caused by the seven affects (or emotions)."

However, there is more to Chinese flower therapy than the beauty of flowers bringing joy. Flower therapy also includes aroma-therapy. A number of Chinese medicinals come from plants which have flowers used in bouquets. For instance, Chrysanthemum flowers (*Ju Hua*, Flos Chrysanthemi Morifolii) are used to calm the liver and clear depressive heat rising to the upper body. The aroma of Chrysanthemum flowers thus also has a salutary, relaxing, and cooling effect on liver depression and depressive heat. Rose (*Mei Gui Hua*, Flos Rosae Rugosae) is used in Chinese medicine to move the qi and quicken the blood. Smelling the fragrance of Roses also does these same things. Other flowers used in Chinese medicine to calm the spirit and relieve stress and irritability are Lily, Narcissus, Lotus flowers, Orchids, and Jasmine. And further, taking a smell of a bouquet of flowers promotes deep breathing, and this, in turn, relieves pent up qi in the chest at the same time as it promotes the flow of qi downward via the lungs.

Thread moxibustion

Thread moxibustion refers to burning extremely tiny cones or "threads" of aged Oriental mugwort directly on top of certain acupuncture points. When done correctly, this is a very simple and effective way of adding yang qi to the body without causing a burn or scar.

To do thread moxa, one must first purchase the finest grade Japanese moxa wool. This is available from Oriental Medical Supplies mentioned above under magnet therapy. It is listed under the name Gold Direct Moxa. Pinch off a very small amount of this loose moxa wool and roll it lightly between the thumb and forefinger. What you want to wind up with is a very loose, very thin thread of moxa smaller than a grain of rice. It is important that this thread not be too large or too tightly wrapped.

Next, rub a very thin film of Tiger Balm or Temple of Heaven Balm on the point to be moxaed. These are camphored Chinese medical salves which are widely available in North American health food stores. Be sure to apply nothing more than the thinnest film of salve. If such a Chinese medicated salve is not available, then wipe the point with a tiny amount of vegetable oil. Stand the thread of moxa up perpendicularly directly over the point to be moxaed. The oil or balm should provide enough stickiness to make the thread stand on end. Light the thread with a burning incense stick. As the thread burns down towards the skin, you will feel more and more heat. Immediately remove the burning thread when you begin to feel the burning thread go from hot to too hot. *Do not burn yourself.* It is better to pull the thread off too soon than too late. In this case, more is not better than enough. (If you do burn yourself, apply some *Ching Wan Hong* ointment. This is a Chinese burn salve which is available at Chinese apothecaries and is truly wonderful for treating all sorts of burns. It should be in every home's medicine cabinet.)

Having removed the burning thread and extinguished it between your two fingers, repeat this process again. To make this process go faster and more efficiently, one can roll a number of threads before starting the treatment. Each time the thread burns down close to the skin, pinch it off the skin and extinguish it *before* it starts to burn you. If you do this correctly, your skin will get red and hot to the touch but you will not raise a blister. Because everyone's skin is different, the first time you do this, only start out with three or four threads. Each day, increase this number until you reach nine to twelve threads per treatment.

This treatment is especially effective for women in their late 30s and throughout their 40s whose spleen and kidney yang qi has already become weak and insufficient. Since this treatment actually adds yang qi to the body, this type of thread moxa fortifies the spleen and invigorates the kidneys, warming yang and boosting the qi. Because the stimuli is not that strong at any given treatment, it must be done every day for a number of days. For women who suffer from PMS with pronounced premenstrual fatigue, loose stools, cold hands and feet, low or no libido, and low back or knee pain accompanied by frequent nighttime urination which ténds to be copious and clear, I recommend beginning this moxibustion just before ovulation, around day 10 in the cycle. It should then be repeated every day up through day one of the period and then suspended. It can be done for several months in a row, but should not usually be done continuously throughout the year, day in and day out.

There are three points which should be moxaed using this supplementing technique. These are:

Qi Hai (Conception Vessel 6)
Guan Yuan (Conception Vessel 4)
Zu San Li (Stomach 36) See p. 117.

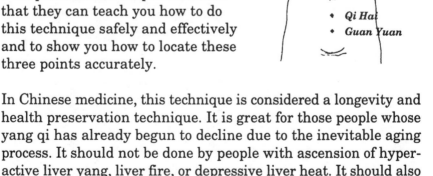

We have already discussed how to locate these three points above. However, I recommend visiting a local professional acupuncturist so that they can teach you how to do this technique safely and effectively and to show you how to locate these three points accurately.

In Chinese medicine, this technique is considered a longevity and health preservation technique. It is great for those people whose yang qi has already begun to decline due to the inevitable aging process. It should not be done by people with ascension of hyperactive liver yang, liver fire, or depressive liver heat. It should also always be done starting from the topmost point and moving downward. This is to prevent leading heat to counterflow upward. If there is any doubt about whether this technique is appropriate for you, please see a professional practitioner for a diagnosis and individualized recommendation.

Chinese Medical Research on PMS

Considerable research has been done in the People's Republic of China on the effects of acupuncture and Chinese herbal medicine on all aspects of PMS. Usually, this research is in the form of a clinical audit. That means that a group of patients with the same diseases, patterns, or major complaints are given the same treatment for a certain period of time. After this time, the patients are counted to see how many were cured, how many got a marked effect, how many got some effect, and how many got no effect. This kind of "outcome-based research" has, up until only very recently, not been considered credible in the West where, for the last 30 years or so, the double-blind, placebo-controlled comparison study has been considered the "gold standard." However, such double-blind, placebo-controlled comparison studies are impossible to design in Chinese medicine and do not, in any case, measure effectiveness in a real-life situation.

Clinical audits, on the other hand, do measure actual clinical satisfaction of real-life patients. Such clinical audits may not exclude the patient's trust and belief in the therapist or the therapy as an important component in the result. However, real-life is not as neat and discreet as a controlled laboratory experiment. If the majority of patients are satisfied with the results of a particular treatment and there are no adverse side effects to that treatment, then that is good enough for the Chinese doctor, and, in my experience, that is also good enough for the vast majority of my patients.

Below are abbreviated translations of several recent research articles published in Chinese medical journals on the treatment of premenstrual breast distention and pain and fibrocystic disease. Many women with premenstrual breast distention and pain also have fibrocystic breasts, and typically, fibrocystic breasts do get worse during the premenstruum These research articles exemplify how Chinese medicine treats one of the most common premenstrual complaints. I think that most women reading these statistics would think that Chinese medicine was worth a try.

"The Pattern Discrimination Treatment of 90 Cases of Menstrual Movement Breast Distention" by Wang Fa-chang & Wang Qu-an, *Shan Dong Zhong Yi Za Zhi (The Shandong Journal of Chinese Medicine)*, #5, 1993, p. 24-25

Menstrual movement, *i.e.*, premenstrual, breast distention and pain is one of the most commonly seen complaints in gynecology departments. The authors of this clinical audit have treated 90 cases of this condition based on pattern discrimination. Of these 90 women, 4 were between 16-20 years old, 11 between 21-25, 20 between 26-30, 21 between 31-35, 20 between 36-40, 5 between 41-45, 7 between 46-50, and 2 cases were more than 50 years old. The course of these women's disease was from one half year to 20 years.

1. Simultaneous liver depression with damp heat pattern

The main symptoms of this pattern are premenstrual chest oppression, heart vexation and easy anger, breast distention and pain, a dry mouth, vexatious heat of the chest and epigastrium, lower abdominal aching and pain, possible vaginal itching or excessive, yellow-colored vaginal discharge, a bowstring, rapid pulse, and red tongue with thin, yellow fur. The treatment principles were to course the liver and resolve depression, clear heat and disinhibit dampness. The formula consisted of a combination of *Dan Zhi Xiao Yao San* (Moutan & Gardenia Rambling Powder), *Yi Huang Tang* (Change Yellow [Discharge] Decoction), and *San Miao San* (Three Wonders Powder) plus Rhizoma Cyperi Rotundi (*Xiang Fu*).

2. Simultaneous liver depression with blood stasis pattern

The main symptoms of this pattern are premenstrual heart vexation and easy anger, breast distention and pain, occasional nodulation, lower abdominal distention and pain disliking pressure, possible scanty menstruation which does not come smoothly, a dark, purplish menstruate containing clots, a bowstring, slippery pulse, and a purplish, dark tongue with static spots or patches and thin, white fur. The treatment principles were to course the liver and resolve depression, quicken the blood, transform stasis, and stop pain. The formula consisted of *Dan Zhi Xiao Yao San* (Moutan & Gardenia Rambling Powder) combined with *Tao Hong Si Wu Tang* (Persica & Carthamus Four Materials Decoction) plus Pericarpium Citri Reticulatae Viride (*Qing Pi*), Rhizoma Corydalis Yanhusuo (*Yan Hu Suo*), and Tuber Curcumae (*Yu Jin*).

3. Simultaneous liver depression with heart/spleen dual vacuity pattern

The main symptoms of this pattern are premenstrual chest oppression, heart vexation and chaotic thoughts, mild, insidious breast pain or small sensations of distention, heart palpitations, dizziness, loss of sleep, profuse dreaming, lack of strength of the entire body, lassitude of the spirit, diminished appetite, excessive, pasty white vaginal discharge, a bowstring, fine pulse, and a pale tongue with teeth marks on its border and thin, white fur. The treatment principles were to course the liver and resolve depression, fortify the spleen and harmonize the stomach, nourish the heart and quiet the spirit. The formula consisted of *Dan Shen Gui Pi Tang* (Salvia Restore the Spleen Decoction) plus Rhizoma Cyperi Rotundi (*Xiang Fu*) and Tuber Curcumae (*Yu Jin*).

133

4. Liver/kidney insufficiency pattern

The main symptoms of this pattern are premenstrual chest oppression, heart vexation and chaotic thoughts, mild, insidious breast pain, dizziness, tinnitus, low back pain, weakness of the extremities, lack of strength, a deep, bowstring pulse, and a pale tongue with scanty fur. The treatment principles were to course the liver and fortify the spleen, supplement and boost the liver and kidneys. The formula consisted of *Dan Zhi Xiao Yao San* (Moutan & Gardenia Rambling Powder) plus Cortex Eucommiae Ulmoidis (*Du Zhong*), Radix Dipsaci (*Chuan Xu Duan*), Ramulus Loranthi Seu Visci (*Sang Ji Sheng*), Cornu Degelatinum Cervi (*Lu Jiao Shuang*), Fructus Corni Officinalis (*Shan Zhu Yu*), and Semen Cuscutae (*Tu Si Zi*).

5. Simultaneous liver depression with *chong* and *ren* vacuity cold pattern

The main symptoms of this pattern are premenstrual heart vexation and chaotic thoughts, lassitude of the spirit, breast distention and pain, insidious lower abdominal pain with a cool sensation, a fine, slow pulse, and a pale tongue with thin, white fur. The treatment principles were to course the liver and resolve depression, cherish the palace (*i.e.*, uterus) and scatter cold. The formula consisted of *Dan Zhi Xiao Yao San* (Moutan & Gardenia Rambling Powder) plus Radix Linderae Strychnifoliae (*Wu Yao*), Rhizoma Cyperi Rotundi (*Xiang Fu*), stir-fried Fructus Foeniculi Vulgaris (*Xiao Hui Xiang*), and stir-fried Folium Artemisiae Argyii (*Ai Ye*).

One course of treatment consisted of three bags of the above formula administered during the woman's premenstruum, one bag being brewed as a "tea" and taken each day. Complete cure was defined as disappearance of such symptoms as premenstrual chest oppression, heart vexation and chaotic thoughts, breast distention and pain, etc. with reduction or disappearance of nodulations and lumps in the breasts within three courses of treatment, *i.e.*, three menstrual cycles. Marked improvement consisted of reduction in such symptoms as premenstrual chest oppression, heart vexation and chaotic thoughts, breast distention and pain, etc. within three courses of treatment. Fair improvement consisted of reduction in the same sorts of symptoms as above in three courses of treatment but recurrence or worsening of these symptoms due to emotional stress. Of the 90 women treated in this study, 57 were cured, 23 were markedly improved, eight experienced fair improvement, and two got no result. Thus the total amelioration rate using this protocol was 97.8%.

"The Treatment of 24 Cases of Fibrocystic Breasts with *Ru Kuai Xiao Tang Jia Wei* (Breast Lump Dispersing Decoction with Added Flavors" by Hou Jian, *Shan Dong Zhong Yi Za Zhi (The Shandong Journal of Chinese Medicine)*, #5, 1993, p. 33

This clinical audit reports on the treatment of 24 cases of fibrocystic breast disease with *Ru Kuai Xiao Tang Jia Wei* from 1989-1991. The age of the women in this study ranged from 23-50 years old, with six cases being between 23-30, 15 between 31-40, and three between 41-50 years of age. Thirteen cases had suffered from this condition for six months or less, five cases from seven months to one year, and six cases for over one year. All these women were married. Treatment used a basic formula which was modified based on pattern discrimination.

1. Liver qi depression & stagnation pattern (13 cases)

The signs and symptoms of this pattern include breast distention and pain which occurred either before the period or got worse with the approach of the period, pain and distention reaching the chest and lateral costal regions, palpable fibrotic tissue and lumps within the breasts but without clearly demarcated borders, lumps may be changeable (*i.e.*, come and go, grow and shrink with the menstrual cycle), lack of ease in emotional affairs, sighing, chest oppression, a darkish pale tongue with thin, white fur, and a bowstring, fine pulse.

2. Phlegm congelation, blood stasis pattern (7 cases)

The signs and symptoms of this pattern include dull breast pain and numbness. However, in prolonged cases, there is piercing pain. In addition there are nodular lumps which do not adhere to the underside of the skin and which are pliable and not hard. Typically, there is physical fatigue, nausea, vomiting of phlegmy saliva, a gloomy (*i.e.*, darkish) tongue with glossy, slimy fur, and a slippery or choppy pulse.

3. *Chong & ren* loss of regulation pattern (4 cases)

The signs and symptoms of this pattern include breast heaviness and pain, many breast lumps spread all over the place occurring before, with, or after menstruation, emotional tension, agitation and easy anger, low back soreness, lack of strength, a pale tongue with white fur, and a soggy or vacuous pulse. This pattern mostly occurs in older women.

Ru Kuai Xiao Tang (the basic formula used in this protocol) consisted of: Fructus Trichosanthis Kirlowii (*Gua Lou*), 15g, uncooked Concha Ostreae (*Mu Li*), 15g, Spica Prunellae Vulgaris (*Xia Gu Cao*), 15g, Thallus Algae (*Kun Bu*), 15g, Herba Sargassii (*Hai Zao*), 15g, Radix Salviae Miltiorrhizae (*Dan Shen*), 15g, Radix Bupleuri (*Chai Hu*), 9g, Tuber Asparagi Cochinensis (*Tian Men Dong*), 9g, Rhizoma Sparganii (*San Leng*), 9g, Rhizoma Curcumae Zedoariae (*E Zhu*), 9g, Folium Citri (*Ju Ye*), 9g, Semen Citri (*Ju He*), 9g, and Rhizoma Pinelliae Ternatae (*Ban Xia*), 9g. These were decocted in water and administered in two divided doses, one bag per day. Treatment was commenced 15 days before the onset of the period, with 12 days equalling one course of treatment. Administration of these medicinals was discontinued during the period itself.

If the pattern was liver qi depression & stagnation, Pericarpium Citri Reticulatae Viride (*Qing Pi*) and Rhizoma Cyperi Rotundi (*Xiang Fu*), 9g @, were added to move the qi and scatter depression. If the pattern was phlegm congelation and blood stasis, the amounts of Concha Ostreae, Thallus Algae, and Radix Salviae Miltiorrhizae were increased up to 30g @ to soften the hard and dispel stasis. If the pattern was *chong* and *ren* loss of regulation, Radix Morindae Officinalis (*Ba Ji Tian*), Cornu Degelatinum Cervi (*Lu Jiao Shuang*), and Retinervus Luffae Cyclindricae (*Si Gua Luo*) were added to secure the kidneys, rectify the *chong*, and free the flow of the network vessels in the breasts.

Complete cure consisted of disappearance of the breast lumps, complete reduction in the aching and pain, and no recurrence on follow-up a half year later. Some improvement was defined as reduction in the size of the lumps and diminishment in the pain and soreness. No results meant that there was no change in either the lumps or the pain. Based on these criteria, in one course of treatment, six women were cured and four got some improvement. In two courses of treatment, three more women were cured and two more got some improvement. In three courses of treatment, three additional women were cured and one more got some improvement. And in four courses of treatment, one more was cured, two more improved, and two got no result. Therefore, the total number of cases cured was 13. The total number of cases improved was nine. And only two women experienced no result. Thus the total amelioration rate was 91.7%.

The author of this article quotes the *Wai Ke Zheng Zong (The True Lineage of External Medicine)* in explaining how this condition comes about:

> Breast aggregation (the traditional Chinese medical name for fibrocystic breasts and breast lumps) consists of nodulations within the breast, their form being like that of an egg. They may be heavy and painful or there may be no pain. The skin (above them) is not changed. These kernels' growth and decline may follow the (growth and decline of) joy and anger. They are mostly

due to worry and anxiety damaging the spleen and irritation and anger damaging the liver with depression binding becoming (nodulation).

"50 Cases Treated for Premenstrual Breast Distention & Pain with *Jie Yu Huo Xue Tang* (Resolve Depression & Quicken the Blood Decoction)" by Gu Si-yun, *Shan Dong Zhong Yi Za Zhi (The Shandong Journal of Chinese Medicine)*, # 6, 1992, p. 27-28

The author of this study begins by saying that premenstrual breast distention is primarily due to liver depression and qi stagnation with subsequent loss of harmony and downbearing of the stomach. Since the breasts are primarily circulated by the liver and stomach channels, qi depression and stagnation affecting these two organs make it difficult for the qi to drain from these channels as they should. Fifty women suffering from premenstrual breast distention and pain were, therefore, treated with the following formula: Radix Bupleuri (*Chai Hu*), 12g, Rhizoma Cyperi Rotundi (*Xiang Fu*), 15g, Radix Ligustici Wallichii (*Chuan Xiong*), 12g, Fructus Citri Aurantii (*Zhi Ke*), 9g, Radix Rubrus Paeoniae Lactiflorae (*Chi Shao*), 12g, Semen Pruni Persicae (*Tao Ren*), 10g, Flos Carthami Tinctorii (*Hong Hua*), 9g, Pericarpium Citri Reticulatae Viride (*Qing Pi*), 10g, Folium Citri (*Ju Ye*), 10g, Fructus Trichosanthis Kirlowii (*Gua Lou*), 15g, Radix Glycyrrhizae (*Gan Cao*), 6g, Radix Salviae Miltiorrhizae (*Dan Shen*), 15g, Tuber Curcumae (*Yu Jin*), 12g, Radix Dioscoreae Oppositae (*Shan Yao*), 12g.

If patients suffered from spleen vacuity, Radix Codonopsitis Pilosulae (*Dang Shen*), Radix Astragali Membranacei (*Huang Qi*), Rhizoma Atractylodis (*Cang Zhu*), Rhizoma Atractylodis Macrocephalae (*Bai Zhu*), and Fructus Amomi (*Sha Ren*) were added. If patients suffered from blood vacuity, Radix Angelicae Sinensis (*Dang Gui*), cooked Radix Rehmanniae (*Shu Di*), and Radix Albus Paeoniae Lactiflorae (*Bai Shao*) were added. If patients suffered from kidney yang vacuity, Cortex Eucommiae Ulmoidis (*Du Zhong*), Semen Cuscutae (*Tu Si Zi*), Radix Dipsaci

(*Xu Duan*), and Herba Epimedii (*Yin Yang Huo*) were added. If patients suffered from kidney yin vacuity, Rhizoma Anemarrhenae Aspheloidis (*Zhi Mu*), uncooked Radix Rehmanniae (*Sheng Di*), Fructus Corni Officinalis (*Shan Zhu Yu*), and Herba Ecliptae Prostratae (*Han Lian Cao*) were added. For liver fire invading the stomach, Fructus Gardeniae Jasminoidis (*Zhi Zi*), Cortex Radicis Moutan (*Dan Pi*), and Pericarpium Citri Reticulatae (*Chen Pi*) were added. For ascendant hyperactivity of liver yang, Ramulus Uncariae Cum Uncis (*Gou Teng*), Concha Margaritiferae (*Zhen Zhu Mu*), Radix Gentianae Scabrae (*Long Dan Cao*), and Flos Chrysanthemi Morifolii (*Ju Hua*) were added. For yin vacuity and yang hyperactivity, Concha Ostreae (*Mu Li*), Gelatinum Corii Asini (*E Jiao*), Tuber Ophiopogonis Japonici (*Mai Dong*), and uncooked Radix Rehmanniae (*Sheng Di*) were added. If there was blood stasis and phlegm congelation, Radix Angelicae Sinensis (*Dang Gui*), Squama Manitis Pentadactylis (*Chuan Shan Jia*), Semen Vaccariae Segetalis (*Wang Bu Liu Xing*), and Rhizoma Sparganii (*San Leng*) were added. These ingredients were decocted in water and one packet of the above herbal medicinals were given per day.

Of the women treated in this study, the oldest was 35 and the youngest was 15 years of age. Twenty women were between the ages of 15 and 20. Eighteen were between the ages of 21 and 30, and 12 were 31 or older. The duration of their disease had lasted from a minimum of six months to a maximum of 10 years, with the average being three years. The above treatment was given for three whole months. At the end of that time, 44 cases or 88% experienced complete cure. Another five cases or 10% experienced some improvement. While only a single case or 2% failed to experience any improvement. Thus the total amelioration rate of the patients participating in this study was 98%.

"The Treatment of 128 Cases of Fibrocystic Breasts" by Mi Yang, *Hu Nan Zhong Yi Za Zhi (The Hunan Journal of Chinese Medicine)*, #1, 1993, p. 47

This clinical audit describes the treatment of 128 cases of fibrocystic breast disease using a formula called *Shen Xiao Gua Lou San*. Sixty-eight cases involved women between the ages of 22-30, 46 cases, 31-40, and 14 cases, 41-55 years of age.

The formula used was *Shen Xiao Gua Lou San* (Magically Dispersing Trichosanthes Powder): Fructus Trichosanthis Kirlowii (*Quan Gua Lou*), 15g, processed Resina Olibani (*Ru Xiang*) and processed Resina Myrrhae (*Mo Yao*), 10g @, Radix Angelicae Sinensis (*Dang Gui*), 12g, and Radix Glycyrrhizae (*Gan Cao*), 6g. These were boiled in 500 ml of water, one packet per day, taken in two divided doses.

If it was possible to feel swelling and lumps within the breast and the emotions were not easy and if there were chest and lateral costal pain and fullness, heart vexation and easy anger, premenstrual breast distention and pain, swelling and lumps which felt achy and painful as if heavy, and pressure caused worsening of the pain, then Radix Bupleuri (*Chai Hu*), Radix Rubrus Paeoniae Lactiflorae (*Chi Shao*), Semen Vaccariae Segetalis (*Wang Bu Liu Xing*), and stir-fried Fructus Citri Aurantii (*Zhi Ke*) were added to this formula. If the breast lumps were stringy or ropy within the breasts or scattered throughout the breasts, if their nature was pliable but tough, menstruation was excessive but pale in color, the four limbs were without strength, and there were dizziness and vertigo, Radix Astragali Membranacei (*Huang Qi*), Radix Codonopsitis Pilosulae (*Dang Shen*), and Fructus Liquidambaris Taiwaniae (*Lu Lu Tong*) were added. If the breasts were swollen and painful and scorching hot, the tongue was red with thin, yellow fur, and the pulse was bowstring and rapid, Flos Lonicerae Japonicae (*Jin Yin Hua*), Fructus Forsythiae Suspensae (*Lian Qiao*), and Herba Taraxaci Mongolici Cum Radice (*Pu Gong Ying*) were added. If the breast lumps were comparatively firm but not hard, if pressure caused aching and pain, and the lumps shifted position when pushed, blast-fried Squama Manitis Pentadactylis (*Chuan Shan Jia*), Spina Gleditschiae Chinensis (*Zao Jiao Ci*), Rhizoma Sparganii (*San Leng*), and Rhizoma Curcumae Zedoariae (*E Zhu*) were added.

Treatment lasted between 30-180 days, with the average being 50 days. Complete cure was defined as disappearance of the lumps. Marked improvement was defined as diminishment of the pain and aching and decrease in the size of the lumps. No result was defined as no diminishment in the pain or aching and no decrease in the size of the lumps. Based on these criteria, 80 cases (62.5%) of the women in this study experienced complete cure; 42 (32.81%) experienced marked improvement; and six cases got no result. Thus the total amelioration rate was 95.31%.

"The Pattern Discrimination Treatment of 100 Cases of Fibrocystic Breasts" by Fang Jian-ping, *Jiang Su Zhong Yi (Jiangsu Chinese Medicine)*, #2, 1993, p. 14

This research report describes the treatment of 100 cases of fibrocystic breast disease based on treating according to a discrimination of patterns. Four patients were between the ages of 15-20; 25 between 21-30; 54 between 31-40; and there were 17 cases between 41-50 years of age. Ninety were married and 10 were unmarried.

1. Liver depression, qi stagnation pattern (45 cases)

The lumps within these women's breasts were large like date pits or chicken eggs. They also presented with emotional lability, heart vexation, and easy anger. The women's menstruation was not easy and there was premenstrual breast heaviness and discomfort, distention and pain. The tongue fur was thin, white or yellow, and the pulse was bowstring. The therapeutic principles were to course the liver and resolve depression, move the qi and scatter nodulation. The formula used was *Xiao Yao San Jia Jian* (Rambling Powder with Additions & Subtractions): vinegar-fried Radix Bupleuri (*Chai Hu*) and stir-fried Fructus Gardeniae Jasminoidis (*Shan Zhi Zi*), 5g @, Radix Albus Paeoniae Lactiflorae (*Bai Shao*), Sclerotium Poriae Cocos (*Fu Ling*), Radix Angelicae Sinensis (*Dang Gui*), Herba Taraxaci Mongolici Cum Radice (*Pu Gong Ying*), Pericarpium Trichosanthis Kirlowii (*Gua Lou Pi*), Pericarpium Citri Reticulatae Viride (*Qing Pi*), Rhizoma Atractylodis Macrocephalae (*Bai Zhu*), and Semen Citri (*Ju He*), 10g @, roasted Rhizoma Zingiberis (*Wei Jiang*) and Radix Glycyrrhizae (*Gan Cao*), 3g @, and processed Squama Manitis Pentadactylis (*Chuan Shan Jia*), 6g.

2. Liver depression, qi vacuity pattern (23 cases)

These women's lumps were divided and scattered or blended into the rest of the tissue and were not easily discernable. They were also movable. Their facial color was sallow white and they had dizziness and vertigo, were exhausted and lacked strength. Their menses were excessive but pale in color, and their tongues were pale with thin, white fur. Their pulses were soggy and fine. The therapeutic principles for this presentation were to course the liver and scatter nodulation, boost the qi and nourish the blood. The formula used was *Si Wu Tang Jia Jian* (Four Materials Decoction with Additions & Subtractions): cooked Radix Rehmanniae (*Shu Di*), Radix Angelicae Sinensis (*Dang Gui*), Radix Albus Paeoniae Lactiflorae (*Bai Shao*), Radix Astragali Membranacei (*Huang Qi*), Sclerotium Poriae Cocos (*Fu Ling*), Tuber Curcumae (*Yu Jin*), Herba Taraxaci Mongolici Cum Radice (*Pu Gong Ying*), and Fructus Liquidambaris Taiwaniae (*Lu Lu Tong*), 10g @, Radix Ligustici Wallichii (*Chuan Xiong*) and Cornu Degelatinum Cervi (*Lu Jiao Shuang*), 5g @, vinegar-fried Radix Bupleuri (*Chai Hu*), 3g, processed Squama Manitis Pentadactylis (*Chuan Shan Jia*), 6g.

3. Liver depression, phlegm nodulation pattern (18 cases)

These women's lumps were disciform or lobular in shape. Their chests, lateral costal regions, and epigastriums were oppressed and distended accompanied by dizziness, a slightly bitter taste in the mouth, abnormal appetite, clots within their menstrual flow, possible loose stools, a pale tongue with white, slimy fur, and a slippery pulse. The therapeutic principles in this case were to course the liver and flush phlegm, soften the hard and scatter nodulation. The formula used was *Lou Feng Fang Tang Jia Jian* (Nidus Vespae Decoction with Additions & Subtractions): Nidus Vespae (*Lou Feng Fang*), Bulbus Cremastrae (*Shan Ci Gu*), processed Squama Manitis Pentadactylis (*Chuan Shan Jia*), and Radix Bupleuri (*Chai Hu*), 6g @, Tuber Curcumae (*Yu Jin*), Pericarpium Citri Reticulatae Viride (*Qing Pi*), Bulbus Fritillariae Thunbergii (*Bei Mu*), Folium Citri (*Ju Ye*), 10g @, processed Rhizoma Cyperi Rotundi (*Xiang Fu*), 12g, and Spica Prunellae Vulgaris (*Xia Gu Cao*), 25g.

4. Qi stagnation, blood stasis pattern (14 cases)

These women's lumps were comparatively firm and like a hard ball in shape. They might also be disciform or lobular. There was aching and pain or pain upon pressure. These lumps had been soft or slippery but had undergone a change. There were clots in these women's menstruate and its color was purplish and dark. Their tongues were purple in color or had purple patches. Their pulses were fine and bowstring. The therapeutic principles in this case were to quicken the blood and dispel stasis, soften the hard and scatter nodulation. The formula used was *Jie Yu Ruan Jian Tang* (Resolve Depression & Soften the Hard Decoction): Radix Angelicae Sinensis (*Dang Gui*), mix-fried Radix Rubrus Paeoniae Lactiflorae (*Chi Shao*), Fructus Tribuli Terrestris (*Bai Ji Li*), Thallus Algae (*Kun Bu*), Herba Sargassii (*Hai Zao*), Cornu Degelatinum Cervi (*Lu Jiao Shuang*), Radix Salviae Miltiorrhizae (*Dan Shen*), and Fructus Crataegi (*Shan Zha*), 10g @, processed Rhizoma Cyperi Rotundi (*Xiang Fu*), processed Squama Manitis

Pentadactylis (*Chuan Shan Jia*), and Tuber Curcumae (*Yu Jin*), 6g
@, Radix Ligustici Wallichii (*Chuan Xiong*), Radix Bupleuri (*Chai Hu*), Pericarpium Citri Reticulatae Viride (*Qing Pi*), and Bulbus
Cremastrae (*Shan Ci Gu*), 5g @, and Herba Taraxaci Mongolici Cum
Radice (*Pu Gong Ying*), 12g. The above medicinals were
administered in decoction internally. At the same time, externally,
Xiao Yan Gao (Disperse Inflammation Plaster) plus *Ru Kuai San*
(Breast Lump Powder, which is composed of Borneolum, *Bing Pian*,
Borax, *Yue Shi*, etc.) were applied above the lumps.

The criteria for success using these protocols were as follows:
Complete cure was defined as disappearance of the lumps,
disappearance of the breast pain, and discontinuance of the
medicinals after three months. Marked improvement was defined
as diminishment of the size of the lumps by half and
disappearance of the breast pain. Some improvement was defined
as diminishment of the size of the lumps by less than half and
reduction in the breast pain. No result was defined as no
reduction in the size of the breast lumps.

Thirty-seven cases of liver depression, qi stagnation experienced
complete cure; six, marked improvement; and two, some
improvement. Sixteen cases of liver depression, qi vacuity
experienced complete cure; five, marked improvement; and two,
some improvement. Eleven cases of qi depression, phlegm
nodulation experienced complete cure; five, marked improvement;
one, some improvement; and one, no result. And eight cases of qi
stagnation, blood stasis experienced complete cure; three, marked
improvement; one, some improvement; and two, no result.
Therefore, the total number of cures was 72; marked
improvement, 19; some improvement, six; and no result, three.
Thus the total amelioration rate was 97%.

Finding a Professional Practitioner of Chinese Medicine

Traditional Chinese medicine is one of the fastest growing holistic health care systems in the West today. At the present time, there are 50 colleges in the United States alone which offer 3-4 year training programs in acupuncture, moxibustion, Chinese herbal medicine, and Chinese medical massage. In addition, many of the graduates of these programs have done postgraduate studies at colleges and hospitals in China, Taiwan, Hong Kong, and Japan. Further, a growing number of trained Oriental medical practitioners have immigrated from China, Japan, and Korea to practice acupuncture and Chinese herbal medicine in the West.

Traditional Chinese medicine, including acupuncture, is a discreet and independent health care profession. It is not simply a technique that can easily be added to the array of techniques of some other health care profession. The study of Chinese medicine, acupuncture, and Chinese herbs is as rigorous as is the study of allopathic, chiropractic, naturopathic, or homeopathic medicine. Previous training in any one of these other systems does not automatically confer competence or knowledge in Chinese medicine. In order to get the full benefits and safety of Chinese medicine, one should seek out professionally trained and credentialed practitioners.

Therefore, below are some abstracts of recent Chinese medical journal articles describing the treatment of PMS with either

Chinese herbal medicine or acupuncture. I present this research for those readers who need "proof" that Chinese medicine does treat PMS effectively.

In the United States of America, recognition that acupuncture and Chinese medicine are their own independent professions has led to the creation of the National Commission for the Certification of Acupuncture & Oriental Medicine (NCCAOM). This commission has created and administers a national board examination in both acupuncture and Chinese herbal medicine in order to insure minimum levels of professional competence and safety. Those who pass the acupuncture exam append the letters Dipl. Ac. (Diplomate of Acupuncture) after their names, while those who pass the Chinese herbal exam use the letters Dipl. C.H. (Diplomate of Chinese Herbs). I recommend that persons wishing to experience the benefits of acupuncture and Chinese medicine should seek treatment in the U.S. only from those who are NCCAOM certified.

In addition, in the United States, acupuncture is a legal, independent health care profession in more than half the states. A few other states require acupuncturists to work under the supervision of MDs, while in a number of states, acupuncture has yet to receive legal status. In states where acupuncture is licensed and regulated, the names of acupuncture practitioners can be found in the *Yellow Pages* of your local phone book or through contacting your State Department of Health, Board of Medical Examiners, or Department of Regulatory Agencies. In states without licensure, it is doubly important to seek treatment only from NCCAOM diplomates.

When seeking a qualified and knowledgeable practitioner, word of mouth referrals are important. Satisfied patients are the most reliable credential a practitioner can have. It is appropriate to ask the practitioner for references from previous patients treated for the same problem. It is best to work with a practitioner who communicates effectively enough for the patient to feel understood and for the Chinese medical diagnosis and treatment plan to make sense. In all cases, a professional practitioner of Chinese medicine should be able and willing to give a written traditional Chinese diagnosis of the patient's pattern upon request.

For further information regarding the practice of Chinese medicine and acupuncture in the United States and for referrals to local professional associations and practitioners in the United States, prospective patients may contact:

National Commission for the Certification of Acupuncture & Oriental Medicine
P.O. Box 97075
Washington DC 20090-7075
Tel: (202) 232-1404
Fax: (202) 462-6157

The National Acupuncture & Oriental Medicine Alliance
14637 Starr Rd, SE
Olalla, WA 98357
Tel: (206) 851-6895
Fax: (206) 728-4841
E mail: 76143.2061@compuserve.com

The American Association of Oriental Medicine
433 Front St.
Catasauqua, PA 18032-2506
Tel: (610) 433-2448
Fax: (610) 433-1832

Learning More About Chinese Medicine

For more information on Chinese medicine in general, see:

The Web That Has No Weaver: Understanding Chinese Medicine by Ted Kaptchuk, Congdon & Weed, NY, 1983. This is the best overall introduction to Chinese medicine for the serious lay reader. It has been a standard since it was first published over a dozen years ago and it has yet to be replaced.

Chinese Secrets of Health & Longevity by Bob Flaws, Sound True, Boulder, CO, 1996. This is a six tape audiocassette course introducing Chinese medicine to laypeople. It covers basic Chinese medical theory, Chinese dietary therapy, Chinese herbal medicine, acupuncture, *qi gong*, *feng shui*, deep relaxation, lifestyle, and more.

Fundamentals of Chinese Medicine by the East Asian Medical Studies Society, Paradigm Publications, Brookline, MA, 1985. This is a more technical introduction and overview of Chinese medicine intended for professional entry level students.

Traditional Medicine in Contemporary China by Nathan Sivin, Center for Chinese Studies, University of Michigan, Ann Arbor, 1987. This book discusses the development of Chinese medicine in China in the last half century as well as introducing all the basic concepts of Chinese medical theory and practice.

Rooted in Spirit: The Heart of Chinese Medicine by Claude Larre & Elisabeth Rochat de la Vallée, trans. by Sarah Stang, Station Hill Press, NY, 1995. This book explains the central concepts of Chinese medicine from a decidely spiritual point of view. Essentially, it is commentary on the eight chapter of the *Nei Jing Ling Shu (Inner Classic: Spiritual Pivot)*.

In the Footsteps of the Yellow Emperor: Tracing the History of Traditional Acupuncture by Peter Eckman, Cypress Book Company, San Francisco, 1996. This book is a history of Chinese medicine and especially acupuncture. In it, the author traces how acupuncture came to Europe and America from China, Hong Kong, Taiwan, Japan, and Korea in the early and middle part of this century. Included are nontechnical discussions of basic Chinese medical theory and concepts.

Knowing Practice: The Clinical Encounter of Chinese Medicine by Judith Farquhar, Westview Press, Boulder, CO, 1994. This book is a more scholarly approach to the recent history of Chinese medicine in the People's Republic of China as well as an introduction to the basic methodology of Chinese medical practice. Although written by an academic sinologist and not a practitioner, it nonetheless contains many insightful and perceptive observations on the differences between traditional Chinese and modern Western medicines.

Imperial Secrets of Health and Longevity by Bob Flaws, Blue Poppy Press, Inc., Boulder, CO, 1994. This book includes a section on Chinese dietary therapy and generally introduces the basic concepts of good health according to Chinese medicine.

Chinese Herbal Remedies by Albert Y. Leung, Universe Books, NY, 1984. This book is about simple Chinese herbal home remedies.

Legendary Chinese Healing Herbs by Henry C. Lu, Sterling Publishing, Inc., NY, 1991. This book is a fun way to begin learning about Chinese herbal medicine. It is full of interesting and entertaining anecdotes about Chinese medicinal herbs.

The Mystery of Longevity by Liu Zheng-cai, Foreign Languages Press, Beijing, 1990. This book is also about general principles and practice promoting good health according to Chinese medicine.

For more information on Chinese gynecology, see:

Breast Health Naturally with Chinese Medicine by Honora Lee Wolfe, Blue Poppy Press, Boulder, CO, 1997. This book is an introduction to Chinese medical theory in terms of breast diseases written by a professional acupuncturist for nonprofessional women readers.

Menopause, A Second Spring: Make A Smooth Transition with Traditional Chinese Medicine by Honora Lee Wolfe, Blue Poppy Press, Boulder, CO, 1995. Written by the same author as the above book, this is a basic introduction to Chinese medicine and how it diagnoses and treats perimenopausal disorders, including osteoporosis.

Endometriosis, Infertility and Traditional Chinese Medicine by Bob Flaws, Blue Poppy Press, Boulder, CO, 1996. Similar to the above two books in conception and tone, this book deals with the Chinese medical diagnosis and treatment of endometriosis and infertility in an easy to understand way.

A Handbook of Menstrual Diseases in Chinese Medicine by Bob Flaws, Blue Poppy Press, Boulder, CO, 1997. This is a comprehensive professional clinical manual on the diagnosis and treatment of dozens of menstrual and premenstrual complaints with both Chinese herbal medicine and acupuncture.

A Handbook of Traditional Chinese Gynecology by the Zhejiang College of Chinese Medicine, Blue Poppy Press, Boulder, CO, 1995. This is also a professional clinical manual covering the diagnosis and treatment of menstrual diseases, abnormal vaginal discharge diseases, gestational and birthing diseases, postpartum diseases, and a number of so-called miscellaneous diseases, such as mastitis, uterine prolapse, and infertility.

Concise Traditional Chinese Gynecology by the Nanjing College of Chinese Medicine, Jiangsu Science & Technology Publishing House, Nanjing, 1988. This is a shorter, more condensed clinical manual on basic Chinese gynecology intended for professional readers.

The English-Chinese Encyclopedia of Practical Traditional Chinese Medicine, Gynecology by Xuan Jia-sheng *et al.*, Higher Education Press, Beijing, 1990. This is another professional entry level text on Chinese gynecology covering comparable material to the above two titles.

For more information on Chinese dietary therapy, see:

The Dao of Healthy Eating According to Traditional Chinese Medicine by Bob Flaws, Blue Poppy Press, Boulder, CO, 1997. This book is a layperson's primer on Chinese dietary therapy. It includes detailed sections on the clear, bland diet as well as sections on chronic candidiasis and allergies.

Prince Wen Hui's Cook: Chinese Dietary Therapy by Bob Flaws & Honora Lee Wolfe, Paradigm Publications, Brookline, MA, 1983. This book is an introduction to Chinese dietary therapy. Although some of the information it contains is dated, it does give the Chinese medicinal descriptions of most foods commonly eaten in the West.

The Book of Jook: Chinese Medicinal Porridges, A Healthy Alternative to the Typical Western Breakfast by Bob Flaws, Blue Poppy Press, Boulder, CO, 1995. This book is specifically about Chinese medicinal porridges made with very simple combinations of Chinese medicinal herbs.

The Tao of Nutrition by Maoshing Ni, Union of Tao and Man, Los Angeles, 1989

Harmony Rules: The Chinese Way of Health Through Food by Gary Butt & Frena Bloomfield, Samuel Weiser, Inc., York Beach, ME, 1985

Chinese System of Food Cures: Prevention & Remedies by Henry C. Lu, Sterling Publishing Co., Inc., NY, 1986

A Practical English-Chinese Library of Traditional Chinese Medicine: Chinese Medicated Diet ed. by Zhang En-qin, Shanghai College of Traditional Chinese Medicine Publishing House, Shanghai, 1990

Eating Your Way to Health — Dietotherapy in Traditional Chinese Medicine by Cai Jing-feng, Foreign Languages Press, Beijing, 1988

Chinese Medical Glossary

Chinese medicine is a system unto itself. Its technical terms are uniquely its own and cannot be reduced to the definitions of Western medicine without destroying the very fabric and logic of Chinese medicine. Ultimately, because Chinese medicine was created in the Chinese language, Chinese medicine is best and really only understood in that language. Nevertheless, as Westerners trying to understand Chinese medicine, we must translate the technical terms of Chinese medicine in English words. If some of these technical translations sound at first peculiar and their meaning is not immediately transparent, this is because no equivalent concepts exist in everyday English.

In the past, some Western authors have erroneously translated technical Chinese medical terms using Western medical or at least quasi-scientific words in an attempt to make this system more acceptable to Western audiences. For instance, the words tonify and sedate are commonly seen in the Western Chinese medical literature even though, in the case of sedate, its meaning is 180° opposite to the Chinese understanding of the word *xie*. *Xie* means to drain off something which has pooled and accumulated. That accumulation is seen as something excess which should not be lingering where it is. Because it is accumulating somewhere where it shouldn't, it is impeding and obstructing whatever should be moving to and through that area. The word sedate comes from the Latin word *sedere*, to sit. Therefore, the word sedate means to make something sit still. In English, we get the word sediment from this same root. However, the Chinese *xie* means draining off which is sitting somewhere erroneously. Therefore, to think that one is going to sedate what is already sitting is a great mistake in understanding the clinical implication and application of this technical term.

Therefore, in order to preserve the integrity of this system while still making it intelligible to English language readers, I have appended the following glossary of Chinese medical technical terms. The terms themselves are based on Nigel Wiseman's *English-Chinese Chinese-English Dictionary of Chinese Medicine* published by the Hunan Science & Technology Press in Changsha, Hunan, People's Republic of China in 1995. Dr. Wiseman is, I believe, the greatest Western scholar in terms of the translation of Chinese medicine into English. As a Chinese reader myself, although I often find Wiseman's terms awkward sounding at first, I also think they convey most accurately the Chinese understanding and logic of these terms.

Acquired essence: Essence manufactured out of the surplus of qi and blood in turn created out of the refined essence of food and drink

Acupoints: Those places on the channels and network vessels where qi and blood tend to collect in denser concentrations, and thus those places where the qi and blood in the channels are especially available for manipulation

Acupuncture: The regulation of qi flow by the stimulation of certain points located on the channels and network vessels achieved mainly by the insertion of fine needles into these points

Aromatherapy: Using various scents and smells to treat and prevent disease

Ascendant hyperactivity of liver yang: Upwardly out of control counterflow of liver yang due to insufficient yin to hold it down in the lower part of the body

Bedroom taxation: Fatigue or vacuity due to excessive sex

Blood: The red colored fluid which flows in the vessels and nourishes and constructs the tissues of the body

Blood stasis: Also called dead blood, malign blood, and dry blood, blood stasis is blood which is no longer moving through the vessels as it should. Instead it is precipitated in the vessels like silt in a river. Like silt, it then obstructs the free flow of the blood in the vessels and also impedes the production of new or fresh blood.

Blood vacuity: Insufficient blood manifesting in diminished nourishment, construction, and moistening of body tissues

Bowels: The hollow yang organs of Chinese medicine

Central qi: Also called the middle qi, this is synonymous with the spleen-stomach qi

Channels: The main routes for the distribution of qi and blood, but mainly qi

Chong **&** *ren***:** Two of the eight extraordinary vessels which act as reservoirs for all the other channels and vessels of the body. These two govern women's menstruation, reproduction, and lactation in particular.

Clear: The pure or clear part of food and drink ingested which is then turned into qi and blood

Counterflow: An erroneous flow of qi, usually upward but sometimes horizontally as well

Damp heat: A combination of accumulated dampness mixed with pathological heat often associated with sores, abnormal vaginal discharges, and some types of menstrual and body pain

Dampness: A pathological accumulation of body fluids

Decoction: A method of administering Chinese medicinals by boiling these medicinals in water, removing the dregs, and drinking the resulting medicinal liquid

Depression: Stagnation and lack of movement, as in liver depression qi stagnation

Depressive heat: Heat due to enduring or severe qi stagnation which then transforms into heat

Drain: To drain off or away some pathological qi or substance from where it is replete or excess

Essence: A stored, very potent form of substance and qi, usually yin when compared to yang qi, but can be transformed into yang qi

Five phase theory: A ancient Chinese system of correspondences dividing up all of reality into five phases of development which then mutually engender and check each other according to definite sequences

Heat toxins: A particularly virulent and concentrated type of pathological heat often associated with purulence (*i.e.*, pus formation), sores, and sometimes, but not always, malignancies

Heliotherapy: Exposure of the body to sunlight in order to treat and prevent disease

Hydrotherapy: Using various baths and water applications to treat and prevent disease

Lassitude of the spirit: A listless or apathetic affect or emotional demeanor due to obvious fatigue of the mind and body

Life gate fire: Another name for kidney yang or kidney fire, seen as the ultimate source of yang qi in the body

Magnet therapy: Applying magnets to acupuncture points to treat and prevent disease

Moxibustion: Burning the herb Artemisia Argyium on, over, or near acupuncture points in order to add yang qi, warm cold, or promote the movement of the qi and blood

Network vessels: Small vessels which form a net-like web insuring the flow of qi and blood to all body tissues

Phlegm: A pathological accumulation of phlegm or mucus congealed from dampness or body fluids

Qi: Activity, function, that which moves, transforms, defends, restrains, and warms

Portals: Also called orifices, the openings of the sensory organs and the opening of the heart through which the spirit makes contact with the world outside

Qi mechanism: The process of transforming yin substance controlled and promoted by the qi, largely synonymous with the process of digestion

Qi vacuity: Insufficient qi manifesting in diminished movement, transformation, and function

Repletion: Excess or fullness, almost always pathological

Seven star hammer: A small hammer with needles embedded in its head used to stimulate acupoints without actually inserting needles

Spirit: The accumulation of qi in the heart which manifests as consciousness, sensory awareness, and mental-emotional function

Stagnation: Non-movement of the qi, lack of free flow, constraint

Supplement: To add to or augment, as in supplementing the qi, blood, yin, or yang

Turbid: The yin, impure, turbid part of food and drink which is sent downward to be excreted as waste

Vacuity: Emptiness or insufficiency, typically of qi, blood, yin, or yang

Vacuity cold: Obvious signs and symptoms of cold due to a lack or insufficiency of yang qi

Vacuity heat: Heat due to hyperactive yang in turn due to insufficient controlling yin

Vessels: The main routes for the distribution of qi and blood, but mainly blood

Viscera: The sold yin organs of Chinese medicine

Yin: In the body, substance and nourishment

Yin vacuity: Insufficient yin substance necessary to both nourish, control, and counterbalance yang activity

Yang: In the body, function, movement, activity, transformation

Yang vacuity: Insufficient warming and transforming function giving rise to symptoms of cold in the body

Bibliography

Chinese language sources

"A Review of the Chinese Medical Literature on Climacteric Syndrome", Yao Shi-an, *Zhong Yi Za Zhi (Journal of Chinese Medicine)*, #2, 1994, p. 112-114

"A Study on the Treatment of Primary Dysmenorrhea with *Jia Wei Mo Jie Tang* (Added Flavors Myrrh & Dragon's Blood Decoction) and Its Effect on Prostaglandins & Related Factors)", Zhu Nan-sun *et al.*, *Zhong Yi Za Zhi (Journal of Chinese Medicine)*, #2, 1994, p. 99-101

Bai Ling Fu Ke (Bai-ling's Gynecology), Han Bai-ling, Heilongjiang People's Press, Harbin, 1983

Cheng Dan An Zhen Jiu Xuan Ji (Cheng Dan-an's Selected Acupuncture & Moxibustion Works), ed. by Cheng Wei-fen *et al.*, Shanghai Science & Technology Press, Shanghai, 1986

Chu Zhen Zhi Liao Xue (A Study of Acupuncture Treatment), Li Zhong-yu, Sichuan Science & Technology Press, Chengdu, 1990

"Clinical Experiences in the Treatment of 120 Cases of Mammary Neoplasia with *Ru Tong Ling* (Breast Pain Efficacious [Remedy])", Ye Xiu-min & Zhang Geng-yang, *Tian Jin Zhong Yi (Tianjin Chinese Medicine)*, #3, 1994, p. 6

Dong Yuan Yi Ji (Dong-yuan's Collected Medical Works), ed. by Bao Zheng-fei *et al.*, People's Health & Hygiene Press, Beijing, 1993

"Experiences in the Treatment of Chronic Fibrocystic Breast Disease", Yang Hui-an, *Tian Jin Zhong Yi (Tianjin Chinese Medicine)*, #6, 1993, p. 9

Fu Ke Bing (Gynecological Diseases), California Certified Acupuncturists Association, Oakland, CA, 1988

Fu Ke Bing Liang Fang (Fine Formulas for Gynecological Diseases), He Yuan-lin & Jiang Chang-yun, Yunnan University Press, Chongqing, 1991

Fu Ke Lin Chuan Jing Hua (The Clinical Efflorescence of Gynecology), Wang Bu-ru & Wang Qi-ming, Sichuan Science & Technology Press, Chengdu, 1989

Fu Ke San Bai Zheng (Three Hundred Gynecological Conditions), Liu Lan-fang & Liu Dian-gong, Jiangxi Science & Technology Press, 1989

Fu Ke Yu Chi (The Jade Ruler of Gynecology), Shen Jin-ao, Shanghai Science & Technology Press, Shanghai, 1983

Fu Ke Zheng Zhi (Gynecological Patterns & Treatments), Sun Jiu-ling, Hebei People's Press, 1983

Fu Qing Zhu Nu Ke (Fu Qing-zhu's Gynecology), Fu Qing-zhu, Shanghai People's Press, Shanghai, 1979; available in English, trans. by Yang Shou-zhong & Liu Da-wei, Blue Poppy Press, Boulder, CO, 1992

Fu Ren Da Quan Liang Fang (A Great Compendium of Fine Formulas for Women), Chen Ze-ming, People's Government Press, Beijing, 1985

Gu Qin Fu Ke Zhen Jiu Miao Fa Da Cheng (A Great Compendium of Ancient & Modern Acupuncture & Moxibustion Miraculous Methods for Gynecology), Liu Ji, Chinese National Chinese Medicine & Medicinals Press, Beijing, 1993

Han Ying Chang Yong Yi Xue Ci Hui (Chinese-English Glossary of Commonly Used Medical Terms), Huang Xiao-kai, People's Health & Hygiene Press, Beijing, 1982

He Zi Huai Nu Ke Jing Yan Ji (A Collection of He Zi-huai's Experiences in Gynecology), ed. by Chen Shao-chun & Lu Zhi, Zhejiang Science & Technology Press, 1982

"Lu De-ming's Experiences Treating Mammary Hyperplasia Disease", Que Hua-fa, *Shang Hai Zhong Yi Yao Za Zhi (Shanghai Journal of Chinese Medicine & Medicinals)*, #2, 1994, p. 6-7

Nan Nu Bing Mi Yan Liang Fang (Secret, Proven, Fine Formulas for Men's & Women's Disease), Du Jie-hui, Beijing Science & Technology Press, Beijing, 1991

Nu Bing Wai Zhi Liang Fang Miao Fa (Fine Formulas & Miraculous Methods for the External Treatment of Women's Diseases), Wang Jin-quan & Cai Yu-hua, Chinese National Chinese Medicine & Medicinals Press, Beijing, 1993

Nu Ke Bai Wen (100 Questions on Gynecology), Qi Chong-fu, Shanghai Ancient Chinese Medical Books Press, Shanghai, 1983

Nu Ke Ji Yao (The Collected Essentials of Gynecology), Yu Yao-feng, People's Government Press, Beijing, 1988

Nu Ke Jing Wei (Profundities from the Gynecological Classics), Lu Guo-zhi & Song Shu-de, Shanxi Science & Technology Press, Xian 1989

Nu Ke Mi Jue Da Quan (A Compendium of Secrets of Success in Gynecology), Chen Liang-fang, Beijing Daily Press, Beijing, 1989

Nu Ke Xian Fang (Immortal Formulas in Gynecology), Fu Shan, aka Fu Qing-zhu, Ancient Chinese Medical Book Press, Beijing, 1989

Nu Ke Yao Zhi (The Essentials of Gynecology), Yu Yo-yuan, Fujian Science & Technology Press, Fuzhou, 1982

Nu Ke Zong Yao (Assembled Essentials of Gynecology), Zhang Shou-qian, Hunan Science & Technology Press, Changsha, 1985

Ru Fang Ji Huan (Breast Diseases & Sufferings), Qiu Si-kang, People's Health & Hygiene Press, Beijing, 1985

Shang Hai Lao Zhong Yi Jing Yan Xuan Bian (A Selected Compilation of Shanghai Old Doctors' Experiences), Shanghai Science & Technology Press, Shanghai, 1984

Shi Yong Zhen Jiu Tui Na Zhi Liao Xue (A Study of Practical Acupuncture, Moxibustion & Tui Na Treatments), Xia Zhi-ping, Shanghai College of Chinese Medicine Press, Shanghai, 1990

Shi Yong Zhong Xi Yi Jie He Fu Chan Ke Zheng Zhi (Proven Treatments in Practical Integrated Chinese-Western Obstetrics & Gynecology), Guo Yuan, Shanxi People's Press, Xian, 1984

Tan Zheng Lun (Treatise on Phlegm Conditions), Hou Tian-yin & Wang Chun-hua, People's Army Press, Beijing, 1989

"The Pattern Discrimination Treatment of 90 Cases of Menstrual Movement Breast Distention", Wang Fa-chang & Wang Qu-an, *Shan Dong Zhong Yi Za Zhi (Shandong Journal of Chinese Medicine)*, #5, 1993, p. 24-25

"The Pattern Discrimination Treatment of 100 Cases of Mammary Hyperplasia", Fang Jian-ping, *Jiang Su Zhong Yi (Jiangsu Chinese Medicine)*, #2, 1993, p. 14

"The Treatment of 50 Cases of Premenstrual Breast Distention & Pain with *Jie Yu Huo Xue Tang* [Resolve Depression & Quicken the Blood Decoction]", Gu Si-yun, *Shan Dong Zhong Yi Za Zhi (Shandong Journal of Chinese Medicine)*, #6, 1992, p. 27-28

"The Treatment of 24 Cases of Mammary Hyperplasia with *Ru Kuai Xiao Tang Jia Wei* [Breast Lump Dispersing Decoction with Added Flavors]", Hou Jian, *Shan Dong Zhong Yi Za Zhi (Shandong Journal of Chinese Medicine)*, #5, 1993, p. 33

"The Treatment of 128 Cases of Mammary Hyperplasia", Mi Yang, *Hu Nan Zhong Yi Za Zhi (Hunan Journal of Chinese Medicine)*, #1, 1993, p. 47

"Use of Basal Body Temperature in Pattern Discrimination for Patients with Infertility and Blocked Menstruation", Xia Gui-cheng, *Shang Hai Zhong Yi Yao Za Zhi (Shanghai Journal of Chinese Medicine & Medicinals)*, #10, 1992, p. 18-19

Wan Shi Fu Ren Ke (Master Wan's Gynecology), Wan Quan, aka Wan Mi-zhai, Hubei Science & Technology Press, 1984

Yi Zong Jin Jian (The Golden Mirror of Ancestral Medicine), Wu Qian *et al.*, People's Health & Hygiene Press, Beijing, 1985

Yu Xue Zheng Zhi (Static Blood Patterns & Treatments), Zhang Xue-wen, Shanxi Science & Technology Press, Xian, 1986

Zhen Jiu Da Cheng (A Great Compendium of Acupuncture & Moxibustion), Yang Ji-zhou, People's Health & Hygiene Press, Beijing, 1983

Zhen Jiu Xue (A Study of Acupuncture & Moxibustion), Qiu Mao-liang *et al.*, Shanghai Science & Technology Press, Shanghai, 1985

Zhen Jiu Yi Xue (An Easy Study of Acupuncture & Moxibustion), Li Shou-xian, People's Health & Hygiene Press, Beijing, 1990

Zhong Guo Min Jian Cao Yao Fang (Chinese Folk Herbal Medicinal Formulas), Liu Guang-rui & Liu Shao-lin, Sichuan Science & Technology Press, Chengdu, 1992

Zhong Guo Zhen Jiu Chu Fang Xue (A Study of Chinese Acupuncture & Moxibustion Prescriptions), Xiao Shao-qing, Ningxia People's Press, Yinchuan, 1986

Zhong Guo Zhong Yi Mi Fang Da Quan (A Great Compendium of Chinese National Chinese Medical Secret Formulas), ed. by Hu Zhao-ming, Literary Propagation Publishing Company, Shanghai, 1992

Zhong Yi Fu Chan Ke Xue (A Study of Chinese Medical Gynecology & Obstetrics), Heilonjiang College of TCM, People's Health and Hygiene Press, Beijing, 1991

Zhong Yi Fu Ke (Chinese Medical Gynecology), Zhu Cheng-han, People's Heath & Hygiene Press, Beijing, 1989

Zhong Yi Fu Ke Lin Chuan Shou Ce (A Clinical Handbook of Chinese Medical Gynecology), Shen Chong-li, Shanghai Science & Technology Press, Shanghai, 1990

Zhong Yi Fu Ke Shou Ce (A Handbook of Chinese Medical Gynecology), Song Guang-ji & Yu Xiao-zhen, Zhejiang Science & Technology Press, Hangzhou, 1984; available in English, fourth, revised edition, trans. by Zhang Ting-liang & Bob Flaws, Blue Poppy Press, Boulder, CO, 1995

Zhong Yi Fu Ke Xue (A Study of Chinese Medical Gynecology), Chengdu College of Chinese Medicine, Shanghai Science & Technology Press, Shanghai, 1983

Zhong Yi Fu Ke Xue (A Study of Chinese Medical Gynecology), Liu Min-ru, Sichuan Science & Technology Press, Chengdu, 1992

Zhong Yi Fu Ke Xue (A Study of Chinese Medical Gynecology), Luo Yuan-qi, Shanghai Science & Technology Press, Shanghai, 1987

Zhong Yi Fu Ke Zhi Liao Shou Ce (A Handbook of Chinese Medical Gynecological Treatment), Wu Shi-xing & Qi Cheng-lin, Shan Xi Science & Technology Press, Xian, 1991

Zhong Yi Hu Li Xue (A Study of Chinese Medical Nursing), Lu Su-ying, People's Health & Hygiene Press, Beijing, 1983

Zhong Yi Lin Chuang Ge Ke (Various Clinical Specialties in Chinese Medicine), Zhang En-qin *et al.*, Shanghai College of TCM Press, Shanghai, 1990

Zhong Yi Ling Yan Fang (Efficacious Chinese Medical Formulas), Lin Bin-zhi, Science & Technology Propagation Press, Beijing, 1991

Zhong Yi Zhi Liao Fu Nu Bing (The Chinese Medical Treatment of Gynecological Diseases), Zhang Jian-xiu, Hebei Science & Technology Press, 1988

Zhong Yi Zi Xue Cong Shu (The Chinese Medicine Self-study Series), Vol. 1, "Gynecology", Yang Yi-ya, Hebei Science & Technology Press, Shijiazhuang, 1987

English language sources

A Barefoot Doctor's Manual, revised & enlarged edition, Cloudburst Press, Mayne Isle, 1977

A Clinical Guide to Chinese Herbs and Formulae, Cheng Song-yu & Li Fei, Churchill & Livingstone, Edinburgh, 1993

A Compendium of TCM Patterns & Treatments, Bob Flaws & Daniel Finney, Blue Poppy Press, Boulder, CO, 1996

A Comprehensive Guide to Chinese Herbal Medicine, Chen Ze-lin & Chen Mei-fang, Oriental Healing Arts Institute, Long Beach, CA, 1992

Arisal of the Clear: A Simple Guide to Healthy Eating According to Traditional Chinese Medicine, Bob Flaws, Blue Poppy Press, Boulder, CO, 1991

A Handbook of Differential Diagnosis with Key Signs & Symptoms, Therapeutic Principles, and Guiding Prescriptions, Ouyang Yi, trans. by C.S. Cheung, Harmonious Sunshine Cultural Center, San Francisco, 1987

Chinese-English Terminology of Traditional Chinese Medicine, Shuai Xue-zhong *et al.*, Hunan Science & Technology Press, Changsha, 1983

Chinese-English Manual of Common-used Prescriptions in Traditional Chinese Medicine, Ou Ming, ed., Joint Publishing Co., Ltd., Hong Kong, 1989

Chinese Herbal Medicine: Formulas & Strategies, Dan Bensky & Randall Barolet, Eastland Press, Seattle, 1990

Chinese Herbal Medicine: Materia Medica, Dan Bensky & Andrew Gamble, second, revised edition, Eastland Press, Seattle, 1993

Chinese Self-massage: The Easy Way to Health, Fan Ya-li, Blue Poppy Press, Boulder, CO, 1996

Chong & Ren Imbalance, Cyclic Management of Menstrual Disorders, Cheng Jing, trans. by C.S. Cheung, Harmonious Sunshine Cultural Center, CA, undated

Concise Traditional Chinese Gynecology, Xia Gui-cheng *et al.*, Jiangsu Science & Technology Press, Nanjing, 1988

English-Chinese Chinese-English Dictionary of Chinese Medicine, Nigel Wiseman, Hunan Science & Technology Press, Changsha, 1995

Fundamentals of Chinese Acupuncture, Andrew Ellis, Nigel Wiseman & Ken Boss, Paradigm Publications, Brookline, MA, 1988

Fundamentals of Chinese Medicine, Nigel Wiseman & Andrew Ellis, Paradigm Publications, Brookline, MA, 1985

Glossary of Chinese Medical Terms and Acupuncture Points, Nigel Wiseman & Ken Boss, Paradigm Publications, Brookline, MA, 1990

Gynecology & Obstetrics: A Longitudinal Approach, ed. by Thomas R. Moore *et al.*, Churchill Livingstone, NY, 1993

Handbook of Chinese Herbs and Formulas, Him-che Yeung, self-published, CA, 1985

"Is Natural Progesterone the Missing Link in Osteoporosis Prevention & Treatment?", J. R. Lee, *Medical Hypotheses*, #35, 1991, p. 316-318

"Menopausal Hormone Replacement Therapy with Continuous Daily Oral Micronized Estradiol and Progesterone", Joel T. Hargrove *et al.*, *Gynecology & Obstetrics*, Vol. 73, #4, April 1989, p. 606-612

Oriental Materia Medica: A Concise Guide, Hong-yen Hsu, Oriental Healing Arts Institute, Long Beach, CA, 1986

"Osteoporosis Reversal: The Role of Progesterone", John R. Lee, *International Clinical Nutrition Review*, Vol. 10, #3, July 1990, p. 384-391

Practical Traditional Chinese Medicine & Pharmacology: Clinical Experiences, Shang Xian-min *et al.*, New World Press, Beijing, 1990

Practical Traditional Chinese Medicine & Pharmacology: Herbal Formulas, Geng Jun-ying, *et al.*, New World Press, Beijing, 1991

"Progesterone and Its Relevance for Osteoporosis", Jerilynn C. Prior, *Osteoporosis*, Vol. 2, #2, March 1993

"Progesterone and the Prevention of Osteoporosis", Jerilynn C. Prior *et al.*, *The Canadian Journal of Ob/Gyn & Women's Health Care*, Vol. 3, #4, 1991, p.178-184

"Progesterone as a Bone-trophic Hormone", J.C. Prior, *Endocrine Reviews*, Vol. 11, #2, 1990, p. 386-398

"Spinal Bone Loss and Ovulatory Disturbances", Jerilynn C. Prior *et al.*, *The New England Journal of Medicine*, Volume 323, #18, November 1, 1990, 12211227

Symptoms and Treatment for Menses and Leukorrhea, Chen Yu-cang, trans. by Hor Ming Lee, Hor Ming Press, Victoria, BC, undated, a translation of *Jing Dai Zheng Zhi (Menstrual & Vaginal Discharge Patterns & Treatments)*

The English-Chinese Encyclopedia of Practical Traditional Chinese Medicine, Vol. 12: Gynecology, Xuan Jia-sheng, ed., Higher Education Press, Beijing, 1990

The Essential Book of Traditional Chinese Medicine, Vol. 2: Clinical Practice, Liu Yan-chi, trans. by Fang Ting-yu & Chen Lai-di, Columbia University Press, NY, 1988

The Merck Manual of Diagnosis & Therapy, 15th edition, ed. by Robert Berkow, Merck Sharp & Dohme Research Laboratories, Rahway, NJ, 1987

The Nanjing Seminars Transcript, Qiu Mao-lian & Su Xu-ming, The Journal of Chinese Medicine, UK, 1985

"The Role of the Liver in Menstrual Disorders", (Rona) Wang Ru & Brian May, *The Pacific Journal of Oriental Medicine,* Australia, #77, p. 10-17

The Treatise on the Spleen & Stomach, Li Dong-yuan, trans. by Yang Shou-zhong, Blue Poppy Press, Boulder, CO 1993

"The Treatment of Fibrocystic Breast Disease with Chinese Herbs and Acupuncture", Deng Hui-ying & Liu Xin-ya, *The Journal of Chinese Medicine,* UK, #52, Sept. 1996, p. 28-30

The Yeast Connection, William G. Crook, Vintage Books, Random House, NY, 1986

The Yeast Syndrome, John Parks Towbridge & Morton Walker, Bantam Books, Toronto, 1988

Traditional Medicine in Contemporary China, Nathan Sivin, University of Michigan, Ann Arbor, 1987

Zang Fu: The Organ Systems of Traditional Chinese Medicine, second edition, Jeremy Ross, Churchill Livingstone, Edinburgh, 1985

Index

OTHER BOOKS ON CHINESE MEDICINE
AVAILABLE FROM BLUE POPPY PRESS
1775 Linden Ave, Boulder, CO 80304
For ordering 1-800-487-9296 PH. 303\447-8372 FAX 303\447-0740

A NEW AMERICAN ACUPUNCTURE by Mark Seem, ISBN 0-936185-44-9

ACUPUNCTURE AND MOXIBUSTION FORMULAS & TREATMENTS by Cheng Dan-an, ISBN 0-936185-68-6,

ACUTE ABDOMINAL SYNDROMES: Their Diagnosis & Treatment by Combined Chinese-Western Medicine by Alon Marcus, ISBN 0-936185-31-7

AGING & BLOOD STASIS: A New Approach to TCM Geriatrics by Yan De-xin, ISBN 0-936185-63-5

AIDS & ITS TREATMENT ACCORDING TO TRADITIONAL CHINESE MEDICINE by Huang Bing-shan, trans. by Fu-Di & Bob Flaws, ISBN 0-936185-28-7

ARISAL OF THE CLEAR: A Simple Guide to Healthy Eating, Bob Flaws, ISBN #-936185-27-9

THE BOOK OF JOOK: Chinese Medicinal Porridges, An Alternative to the Typical Western Breakfast by Bob Flaws, ISBN0-936185-60-0

CHINESE MEDICAL PALMISTRY: Your Health in Your Hand by Zong Xiao-fan & Gary Liscum, ISBN 0-936185-64-3

CHINESE MEDICINAL TEAS: Simple, Proven, Folk Formulas for Common Diseases by Zong & Liscum, ISBN 0-936185-76-7

CHINESE MEDICINAL WINES & ELIXIRS by B. Flaws, ISBN 0-936185-58-9

CHINESE PEDIATRIC MASSAGE THERAPY: A Parent's & Practitioner's Guide to Prevention & Treatment of Childhood Illness by Fan, ISBN 0-936185-54-6

CHINESE SELF-MASSAGE THE- RAPY: The Easy Way to Health by Fan Ya-li ISBN 0-936185-74-0

A COMPENDIUM OF TCM PATTERNS & TREATMENTS by Bob Flaws & Daniel Finney, ISBN 0-936185-70-8

THE DAO OF INCREASING LONGEVITY AND CONSERVING ONE'S LIFE by Anna Lin & Bob Flaws, ISBN 0-936185-24-4

THE DIVINELY RESPONDING CLASSIC: A Translation of the Shen Ying Jing from Zhen Jiu Da Cheng, trans. by Yang & Liu ISBN 0-936185-55-4

DUI YAO: THE ART OF COMBINING CHINESE MEDICINALS by P. Sionneau. trans. by Bernard Côté. ISBN 0-936185-81-3

ENDOMETRIOSIS, INFERTILITY AND TCM: A Laywoman's Guide by Bob Flaws ISBN 0-936185-14-7

EXTRA TREATISES BASED ON INVESTIGATION & INQUIRY: A Translation of Zhu Dan-xi's Ge Zhi Yu Lun, by Yang & Duan, ISBN 0-936185-53-8

FIRE IN THE VALLEY: TCM Diagnosis & Treatment of Vaginal Diseases ISBN 0-936185-25-2

FLESHING OUT THE BONES: The Importance of Case Histories in Chin. Med. trans. by C. Chace. ISBN 0-936185-30-9

FU QING-ZHU'S GYNECOLOGY trans. by Yang and Liu, ISBN 0-936185-35-X

FULFILLING THE ESSENCE: A Handbook of Traditional & Contemporary Treatments for Female Infertility by Bob Flaws, ISBN 0-936185-48-1

GOLDEN NEEDLE WANG LE-TING: A 20th Century Master's Approach to Acupuncture by Yu Hui-chan and Han Fu-ru, trans. by Shuai Xue-zhong, ISBN 0-926185-78-3

A HANDBOOK OF TRADITIONAL CHINESE DERMATOLOGY by Liang, trans. by Zhang & Flaws, ISBN 0-936185-07-4

A HANDBOOK OF TRADITIONAL CHINESE GYNECOLOGY by Zhejiang College of TCM, trans. by Zhang Ting-liang, ISBN 0-936185-06-6 (4nd edit.)

A HANDBOOK OF MENSTRUAL DISEASES IN CHINESE MEDICINE by Bob Flaws ISBN 0-936185-82-1

A HANDBOOK of TCM PEDIATRICS by Bob Flaws, ISBN 0-936185-72-4

A HANDBOOK OF TCM UROLOGY & MALE SEXUAL DYSFUNCTION by Anna Lin, OMD, ISBN 0-936185-36-8

THE HEART & ESSENCE OF DAN-XI'S METHODS OF TREATMENT by Xu Dan-xi, trans. by Yang, ISBN 0-926185-49-X

THE HEART TRANSMISSION OF MEDICINE by Liu Yi-ren; translated by Yang Shou-zhong ISBN 0-936185-83-X

HIGHLIGHTS OF ANCIENT ACUPUNCTURE PRESCRIPTIONS trans. by Wolfe & Crescenz ISBN 0-936185-23-6

How to Have A HEALTHY PREGNANCY, HEALTHY BIRTH with Chinese Medicine by Wolfe, ISBN 0-936185-40-6

HOW TO WRITE A TCM HERBAL FORMULA: A Logical Methodology for the Formulation & Administration of Chinese Herbal Medicine in Decoction by Flaws, ISBN 0-936185-49-X

IMPERIAL SECRETS OF HEALTH & LONGEVITY by Flaws, ISBN 0-936185-51-1

KEEPING YOUR CHILD HEALTHY WITH CHINESE MEDICINE by Bob Flaws, ISBN 0-936185-71-6

Li Dong-yuan's TREATISE ON THE SPLEEN & STOMACH, A Translation of the Pi Wei Lun by Yang Shou-zhong & Li Jian-yong, ISBN 0-936185-41-4

LOW BACK PAIN: Care & Prevention with Chinese Medicine by Douglas Frank, ISBN 0-936185-66-X

MASTER HUA'S CLASSIC OF THE CENTRAL VISCERA by Hua Tuo, ISBN 0-936185-43-0

THE MEDICAL I CHING: Oracle of the Healer Within by Miki Shima, ISBN 0-936185-38-4

MENOPAUSE A Second Spring: Make a Smooth Transition with Chinese Medicine by Wolfe ISBN 0-936185-18-X

PAO ZHI: Introduction to Processing Chinese Medicinals to Enhance Their Therapeutic Effect, Philippe Sionneau, ISBN 0-936185-62-1

PATH OF PREGNANCY, VOL. I, Gestational Disorders by Bob Flaws, ISBN 0-936185-39-2 Vol. II, Postpartum Diseases by Bob Flaws. ISBN 0-936185-42-2

PRINCE WEN HUI'S COOK: Chinese Dietary Therapy by Bob Flaws & Honora Lee Wolfe, ISBN 0-912111-05-4

THE PULSE CLASSIC: A Translation of the Mai Jing by Wang Shu-he, trans. Yang Shou-zhong ISBN 0-936185-75-9

RECENT TCM RESEARCH FROM CHINA, trans. by Charles Chace & Bob Flaws, ISBN 0-936185-56-2

SEVENTY ESSENTIAL TCM FORMULAS FOR BEGINNERS by Bob Flaws, ISBN 0-936185-59-7

SHAOLIN SECRET FORMULAS for Treatment of External Injuries, by De Chan, ISBN 0-936185-08-2

STATEMENTS OF FACT IN TRADITIONAL CHINESE MEDICINE by Bob Flaws, ISBN 0-936185-52-X

STICKING TO THE POINT: A Rational Methodology for the Step by Step Formulation & Administration of an Acupuncture Treatment by Bob Flaws ISBN 0-936185-17-1

THE SYSTEMATIC CLASSIC OF ACUPUNCTURE & MOXIBUSTION (Jia Yi Jing) by Huang-fu Mi, trans. by Yang Shou-zhong and Charles Chace, ISBN 0-936185-29-5

THE TREATMENT OF DISEASE IN TCM, Vol I: Diseases of the Head & Face Including Mental/Emotional Disorders by Philippe Sionneau & Lü Gang, ISBN 0-936185-69-4

THE TREATMENT OF DISEASE IN TCM, Vol. II: Diseases of the Eyes, Ears, Nose, & Throat by Sionneau & Lü, ISBN 0-936185-69-4

THE TREATMENT OF DISEASE, VOL. III: Diseases of the Mouth, Lips, Tongue, Teeth & Gums, by Sionneau & Lü, ISBN 0-936185-79-1

THE TREATMENT OF EXTERNAL DISEASES WITH ACUPUNCTURE & MOXIBUSTION by Yan Cui-lan and Zhu Yun-long, ISBN 0-936185-80-5